Living a Healthy Life

with

Self-Management of *Heart Disease, Arthritis, Diabetes, Asthma, Bronchitis, Emphysema & others*

Chronic Conditions

Second Edition

Kate Lorig, R.N., Dr. P.H.
Halsted Holman, M.D.
David Sobel, M.D.

Diana Laurent, M.P.H.
Virginia González, M.P.H.
Marian Minor, R.P.T., Ph.D.

Contributor: Peg Harrison, M.A., M.S.W., L.C.S.W.

ISBN 0-923521-53-4

Bull Publishing Company
P.O. Box 208
Palo Alto, California 94302-0208
(650) 322-2855
www.bullpub.com

ii
___

Supported by AHCPR Grant HSO 6680 and California State Tobacco-Related Disease Research Program Award 1RT 156

Distributed in the U.S. by: Publishers Group West

Library of Congress Cataloging-in-Publication Data

Living a healthy life with chronic conditions : self-management of heart disease,
arthritis, diabetes, asthma, bronchitis, emphysema & others / Kate Lorig ... [et al.]. —2nd ed.
    p.cm.
  Includes bibliographical references and index.
  ISBN 0-923521-53-4
  1. Chronic diseases—Popular works. 2. Medicine, Popular. I. Lorig, Kate

RC108.L565 2000
616'.044—dc21   00-022528

Publisher: James Bull
Cover Design: Lightbourne Images
Interior Design and Composition: Shadow Canyon Graphics
Illustrations: Publication Services
Editing and Proofreading: Margaret Moore

———————

To David Bull,
who made this book possible

TABLE OF CONTENTS

ACKNOWLEDGMENTS vii

CHAPTER 1
Overview of Self-Management 1

CHAPTER 2
Becoming an Active Self-Manager 15

CHAPTER 3
Finding Resources 27

CHAPTER 4
Understanding Common Symptoms 35

CHAPTER 5
Using Your Mind to Manage Symptoms 63

CHAPTER 6
Exercising for Fun and Fitness 79

CHAPTER 7
Exercising for Flexibility and Strength: Warm-Up/Cool-Down 93

CHAPTER 8
Exercising for Endurance: Aerobic Activities 113

CHAPTER 9
Exercising Tips for People with Specific Chronic Illnesses 131

CHAPTER 10
Communicating 141

CHAPTER 11

Sex and Intimacy 159

CHAPTER 12

Making Your Wishes Known: Advance Directives for Health Care 167

CHAPTER 13

Healthy Eating 177

CHAPTER 14

Managing Your Medicines 205

CHAPTER 15

Understanding Chronic Lung Disease 217

CHAPTER 16

Understanding Heart Disease and High Blood Pressure 241

CHAPTER 17

Understanding Arthritis 261

CHAPTER 18

Understanding Diabetes 271

CHAPTER 19

Planning for the Future: Fears and Reality 293

CHAPTER 20

200+ Helpful Hints 309

INDEX 325

v

ACKNOWLEDGMENTS

Many people have helped us write this book. Among the most important are the first 1000 participants of the Stanford University Chronic Disease Self-Management study. These have been followed by thousands of other course participants in the United States, Australia, New Zealand, Canada, and Great Britain. All of these people, along with our wonderful course leaders, have told us what information they needed and helped us make adjustments as we went along.

There are also many professionals who have assisted us: Susan Kayman, Suephy Chen, Sandra Wilson, Margo Harris, Nancy Brannigan, Jim Phillips, Jean Thompson, Lynne Newcombe, John Lynch, Mary Hobbs, Marty Klein, Nazanin Dashtara, Vivian Vestal, María Hernández-Marin, Richard Rubio, and Laurie Doyle. To all of you, your help has been greatly received. A special thanks to Gloria Samuel, who kept us all on track and put this book together.

Finally, thanks to David Bull to whom this book is dedicated. David was our first publisher and had faith in this project that allowed us to proceed. Without him, there may never have been a book. His son Jim has continued the family tradition with support and encouragement for this second edition.

CHAPTER
1

Overview of Self-Management

1

NOBODY WANTS TO HAVE A CHRONIC LONG-TERM ILLNESS. Unfortunately, most of us will have two or more of these conditions during our lives. This book has been written to help people with chronic illness learn a healthy way to live with a disease. Now, this may seem like a strange concept. How can one have an illness and live a healthy life at the same time? To answer this, we need to look at the consequences of most chronic diseases. These diseases, be they heart disease, diabetes, liver disease, emphysema, or any one of a host of others, cause most people to lose physical conditioning and experience fatigue. In addition, they may cause emotional distress such as frustration, anger, depression, or helplessness. Health is soundness of body and mind, and a healthy life is one which seeks that soundness. Therefore, a healthy way to live with a chronic illness is to work at overcoming the physical and emotional problems caused by the disease. The goal is to achieve the greatest possible physical capability and pleasure from life. That is what this book is all about.

You will not find any miracles or cures in these pages. Rather, you will find hundreds of tips and ideas to make your life easier. This advice comes from physicians, other health professionals, and, most importantly, people like you who have learned to positively manage their illness. Please note that we said *positively* manage. You see, there is no way you can avoid managing a chronic condition. If you do nothing but suffer, this is a management style. If you only take medication, this is another management style. If you choose to be a positive self-manager and take all the best treatments that health care professionals have to offer along with being proactive in your day-to-day management, this will lead you to living a healthy life.

In this chapter, we discuss chronic illness in general as well as point out the most common problems. In addition, we give some guidance on the self-management

Table 1.1 *Differences Between Acute and Chronic Disease*

	Acute Disease	**Chronic Disease**
Beginning	rapid	gradual
Cause	usually one	many
Duration	short	indefinite
Diagnosis	commonly accurate	often uncertain, especially early
Diagnostic Tests	often decisive	often of limited value
Treatment	cure common	cure rare
Role of Professional	select and conduct therapy	teacher and partner
Role of Patient	follow orders	partner of health professionals, responsible for daily management

2

skills that are unique to particular conditions. You will soon see that the problems and skills have much more in common than you might think. The rest of the book deals with the details you will need to master many of the self-management skills.

Chronic Disease

We think of a health problem as being either "acute" or "chronic." Acute health problems usually begin suddenly with a single, easily diagnosed cause, are of short duration, and will respond to a specific treatment such as medication or surgery. For most acute illnesses, a cure with return to normal health is to be expected. For the patient and the doctor there is relatively little uncertainty. One usually knows what to expect. The illness typically has a cycle of getting worse for a while, being treated, and then getting better. Finally, the care of acute illness depends on a health professional's knowledge and experience to find and administer the correct treatment.

Appendicitis is an example of an acute illness, which typically begins rapidly, signaled by nausea and pain in the abdomen. The diagnosis of appendicitis, established by physical examination, leads to surgery for removal of the inflamed appendix. There follows a period of recovery and then a return to normal health.

Chronic illnesses are different. They begin slowly and proceed slowly. For example, a person with long-term arteriosclerosis might have a heart attack or a stroke.

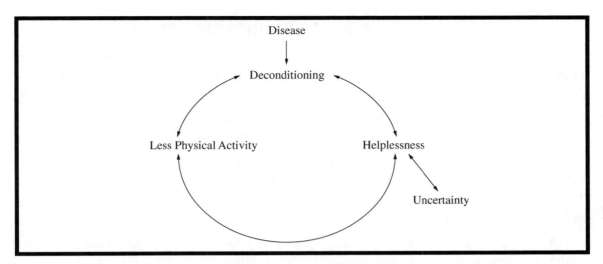

Figure 1.1 *Cycle of Physical Deconditioning and Helplessness*

Most arthritis starts with little annoying twinges that gradually increase. Unlike acute disease, chronic illnesses have multiple causes varying over time and include heredity, lifestyle factors (smoking, lack of exercise, poor diet, stress, etc.), exposure to environmental factors, and physiological factors.

This can be frustrating for those of us who want quick answers. It is difficult for the doctor and the patient when immediate answers aren't available. In some cases, even when diagnosis is rapid, such as in the case of a stroke or heart attack, the long-term effects may be hard to predict. The lack of a regular or predictable pattern in chronic illness is a major characteristic in most chronic illness.

Unlike acute disease, where full recovery is expected, chronic illness usually leads to persistent loss of physical conditioning. Because chronically ill people tire easily, they are unable to accomplish what they once could. They are forced to give up recreational activities like walking, tennis, and golf and chores like shopping, housework, and yard work. This lack of activity accelerates physical deconditioning. At the same time, the loss of physical activity and uncertainty about the future create a sense of helplessness, a feeling that little or nothing can be done to alleviate the situation. Of course, believing nothing can be done is a guarantee that nothing will be done, reinforcing helplessness and perpetuating the vicious cycle. A primary problem of living with chronic illness is dealing with this cycle of physical deconditioning and helplessness (see Figure 1.1).

Table 1.1 summarizes the differences between acute and chronic disease. Throughout this book we examine ways of breaking the cycle and getting away from the problems of physical deconditioning and helplessness which often result from chronic illness.

What Causes a Chronic Disease?

To answer this question, we need to understand how the body operates. As you know, cells are the building blocks of tissues and organs: the heart, lungs, brain, blood, blood vessels, bones, muscles, in fact, everything in the body. For a cell to remain alive and function normally, three things must happen: It must be nourished, receive oxygen, and get rid of waste products. If anything goes wrong with any of these three functions, the cell is diseased. If cells are diseased, the organ or tissue suffers, which may be experienced as limitations in your ability to be active in daily life. The difference in chronic diseases depends on which cells and organs are affected and the processes by which the effect occurs. For example, in a stroke, a blood vessel in the brain becomes blocked or breaks. Oxygen and nutrition are cut off from part of the brain, as a result of which, the parts of your body controlled by the damaged brain cells, such as an arm or a leg or a portion of the face, lose function.

If you have heart disease, several things might happen. For instance, heart attacks occur when the blood vessels supplying blood to the heart muscle become blocked. This is called a *coronary thrombosis*. When this happens, oxygen is cut off, the heart muscle is injured, and pain results. After the injury the heart may be less effective in supplying the rest of your body with oxygen-carrying blood. Because the heart is pumping blood less efficiently through the body, fluid accumulates in tissues, and one experiences shortness of breath.

With bronchitis, asthma, and emphysema, there is either a problem getting oxygen to the lungs, as with bronchitis or asthma, or the lungs cannot effectively transfer oxygen to the blood, as with emphysema. In both cases the body is deprived of oxygen. In diabetes, the pancreas does not produce enough insulin or produces insulin that cannot be used efficiently by the body. Without this insulin the body's cells are not able to use the glucose (sugar) in the blood for energy. In liver and kidney disease, the cells of these organs do not work properly, making it difficult for the body to get rid of waste products.

The basic consequences of these diseases are similar: loss of function due to a reduction in oxygen, accumulation of waste products, or inability of the body to utilize glucose for energy. Loss of function also occurs in arthritis, but for other reasons. In osteoarthritis, cartilage, the tough material found on the ends of bones and as the "disks" between the vertebrae bones of the back, becomes worn, frayed, or displaced, causing pain. We do not know exactly why the cartilage cells begin to weaken or die. But the results are pain and disability.

So far, you can see that all chronic illness starts at a cellular level. But an illness is more than cellular malfunction. It also involves the problems of everyday life, which may include not doing the things you want to do and needing to change your social activities. However, until you get symptoms (shortness of breath, fatigue, pain, etc.) you won't know you have a disease.

Although the biological causes of chronic diseases differ, the problems they cause for patients are similar. For example, most people with chronic disease suffer fatigue and loss of energy. Sleeping problems are not uncommon. In one case there is pain, while in another case there is trouble breathing. Disability, to some extent, is a part of chronic disease. It may be an inability to use your hands well because of arthritis or stroke, or difficulty in walking due to shortness of breath, stroke, arthritis, or diabetes. Sometimes disability is caused by a lack of energy or extreme fatigue.

Another common problem with chronic illness is depression, or just "feeling blue." It is hard to have a cheerful disposition when your condition causes problems that probably won't go away. Along with the depression comes fear and concern for the future. Will I be able to remain independent? If I can't care for myself, who will

5

Chart 1 *Self-Management Problems for Common Chronic Conditions*

Chronic Condition	POSSIBLE PROBLEMS CAUSED BY CHRONIC CONDITIONS				
	Pain	Fatigue	Shortness of Breath	Physical Function	Emotions
Arthritis	X	X		X	X
Asthma and Lung Disease		X	X	X	X
Cancer	X	X		X	X
Chronic Heartburn and Acid Reflux	X				
Chronic Pain	X	X		X	X
Congestive Heart Failure		X	X		X
Diabetes	X	X		X	X
Heart Disease	X	X	X	X	X
Hepatitis	X	X			X
High Blood Pressure					X
HIV Disease (AIDS)	X	X	X	X	X
Inflammatory Bowel Disease	X				X
Irritable Bowel Syndrome	X				X
Kidney Stones	X				
Multiple Sclerosis		X		X	X
Parkinson's Disease		X		X	X
Peptic Ulcer Disease	X				X
Renal Failure		X			X
Stroke		X		X	X

care for me? What will happen to my family? Will I get worse? Disability and depression bring loss of self-esteem.

One of the most important things to learn is that, because of similarities among chronic illnesses, the central management tasks and skills one must learn to live with different chronic illnesses are similar. Besides overcoming physical and emotional problems, you must learn problem-solving skills and how to respond to the trends in your disease. These tasks and skills include developing and maintaining exercise and nutrition programs, managing symptoms, making decisions about when to seek medical help, working effectively with your doctor, using medications and minimizing side effects, finding and using community resources, talking about your illness with family and friends, and, if necessary, changing social activities. Maybe the most important skill of all is learning to respond to your illness on an on-going basis to solve day-to-day problems as they arise. Chart 1 illustrates some of the self-management problems for common chronic conditions.

From this brief introduction, you can see that chronic illnesses have more in common than first meets the eye. In this book, we talk about managing these illnesses. In most of the book, however, we will talk more about the management tasks common across many illnesses. If you have more than one health problem, you need not be confused about how to start. The approaches that work for heart disease will also help with lung disease, arthritis, or a stroke. Start with the problem or condition that bothers you most. Chart 2 outlines some of the management skills that may be needed to deal with disease-specific problems. Some of these skills are also discussed later in the book in the chapters dealing with specific diseases.

Before we discuss management techniques, however, let us talk more about what we mean by self-management.

The Chronic Illness Path

The first responsibility of any chronic disease self-manager is to understand your disease. This means more than learning about what causes the disease and what you can do. It also means observing how the disease and its treatment affect you. Disease is different for each person, and with experience you and your family will become experts at determining the effects of the disease and its treatment. In fact, you are the only person who lives with your disease every day. Therefore, observing your disease and making accurate reports to your health care providers are essential parts of being a good manager. As we mentioned before, most chronic illnesses go up and down in intensity. They do not have a steady path.

The visits on the graph in Figure 1.2 represent Pat's regular follow-up appointments with the doctor or other health professional. Even though the intensity of

Chart 2 *Management Skills for Dealing with Common Chronic Conditions*

MANAGEMENT SKILLS

CHRONIC CONDITION	Pain Management	Fatigue Management	Breathing Techniques	Relaxation and Managing Emotions	Nutrition	Exercise	Medications	Other Management Tools
Arthritis	X	X		X	X	X	X	• Use of assistive devices • Appropriate use of joints • Use of cold/heat • Pacing of activities
Asthma and Lung Disease		X	X	X		X	X	• Use of inhalers and peak flow meters • Avoid triggers
Cancer	X	X		X	X		X	• Varies with site of the cancer • Managing surgery, radiation, and chemotherapy
Chronic Pain	X	X		X		X	X	• Pacing of activities • Specific exercises • Adjust ergonomics and activities
Congestive Heart Failure		X	X	X	X	X	X	• Monitoring of daily weight • Sodium/salt restriction
Diabetes	X	X		X	X	X	X	• Home blood glucose monitoring • Insulin injection • Foot care • Regular eye (retinal) exams

(continues)

7

Chart 2 (continued) *Management Skills for Dealing with Common Chronic Conditions*

MANAGEMENT SKILLS

CHRONIC CONDITION	Pain Management	Fatigue Management	Breathing Techniques	Relaxation and Managing Emotions	Nutrition	Exercise	Medications	Other Management Tools
Heartburn and Acid Reflux					X		X	• Avoid stomach irritants (e.g., coffee, alcohol, aspirin, nonsteroidal anti-inflammatory medications) • Elevation of bed
Heart Disease	X	X	X	X	X	X	X	• Know and watch for warning signs of heart attack
Hepatitis	X	X		X	X		X	• Avoid use of alcohol, IV drugs, medications toxic to liver • Preventing spread of infection (e.g., for hepatitis B and C, safer sex practices, hygiene
High Blood Pressure				X	X	X	X	• Home blood pressure monitoring • Sodium/salt restriction
HIV Disease (AIDS)	X	X	X	X	X	X	X	• Preventing spread of infection (e.g., safer sex practices, hygiene) • Watch for signs of early infection • Avoid IV drugs

Chart 2 (continued) *Management Skills for Dealing with Common Chronic Conditions*

MANAGEMENT SKILLS

CHRONIC CONDITION	Pain Management	Fatigue Management	Breathing Techniques	Relaxation and Managing Emotions	Nutrition	Exercise	Medications	Other Management Tools
Inflammatory Bowel Disease	X			X	X		X	
Irritable Bowel Syndrome	X			X	X		X	
Kidney Stones	X				X		X	• Maintain fluid intake • Avoid calcium or oxalates, depending on type of stone
Multiple Sclerosis		X		X		X	X	• Management of incontinence • Management of mobility
Parkinson's Disease		X		X		X	X	• Mobility
Peptic Ulcer Disease	X			X	X		X	• Avoid stomach irritants (e.g., coffee, alcohol, aspirin, nonsteroidal anti-inflammatory medications)
Renal Failure		X		X	X		X	• Dialysis
Stroke		X		X	X	X	X	• Use of assistive devices

9

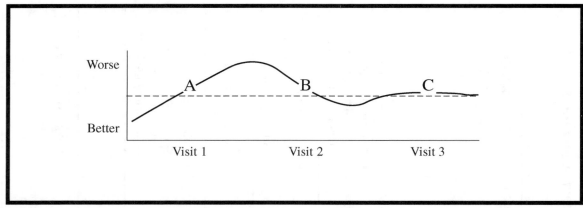

Figure 1.2 *Illness Path*

10

Pat's symptoms are at the same level for all three visits, what has happened in the time between the appointments can mean entirely different things when the health care team is evaluating whether to maintain or change treatment. In the case of the first visit, the symptoms are getting better, so keeping the treatment stable or even lessening it may be in order; in the case of the second visit, things seem to be getting worse, so additional treatment may be the choice. In the case of the third visit, things have been stable for a while, so maintaining treatment may be the best treatment option.

Your experience and understanding, communicated clearly to the physician, are often the best indicators of the path's course, and skilled clinicians commonly depend on them. In fact, if the clinician encourages and facilitates learning by the patient and the patient responds by participating in decisions, a partnership is born. To be most effective, self-management of chronic illness requires such a partnership.

When you develop a chronic illness, you become more aware of your body. Minor symptoms which were formerly ignored may now cause concerns. For example, is this chest pain a signal of a heart attack? Is this pain in my knee a sign that the arthritis has spread? There are no simple reassuring answers to apply to all patients. Nor is there a fail-safe way of sorting out serious signals from minor temporary symptoms that can be ignored.

It is helpful to understand the natural rhythms of your chronic illness. In general, symptoms should be checked out with your doctor if they are *unusual, severe, persistent,* or *occur after starting a new medication.*

Throughout this book, we give some specific examples of what actions to take if you experience certain symptoms. But this is where your partnership with your health care provider becomes most critical. He or she can help guide you in responding to specific problems or symptoms. Self-management does not mean going it alone. Get help or advice when you are concerned or uncertain.

In terms of what has just been said, self-management may seem like a simple enough term. Both at home and in the business world, managers direct the show. They don't do everything themselves; they work with others, including consultants, to get the job done. What makes them managers is that they are responsible for making the decisions and making sure these decisions are carried out.

As a manager of your illness, your job is much the same. You gather information and hire a consultant, or a team of consultants consisting of your physician and other health professionals. Once they have given you their best advice, it is up to you to follow through. All chronic illness needs day-to-day management. We have all noticed that some people with severe physical problems get on well while others with lesser problems seem to give up on life. The difference is often management style.

Managing a chronic illness, like managing a family or a business, is a complex undertaking. There are many twists, turns, and midcourse corrections. By learning self-management skills, you can ease the problems of living with your condition.

The key to success in any undertaking is first deciding what you want to do, second, deciding how you are going to do it, and, finally, learning a set of skills and practicing them until they have been mastered. These tasks are all based on learning skills and mastering them. Success in chronic disease self-management is the same. In fact, mastering such skills is one of the most important tasks of later life.

We will describe hundreds of skills and strategies to help relieve the problems caused by chronic illness. We do not expect you to do all of them. Pick and choose. Experiment. Set your own goals. *What* you do may not be as important as the sense of confidence and control that comes from successfully doing something you *want* to do. However, we have learned that knowing the skills is not enough. We need a way of incorporating these skills into our daily lives. Whenever we try a new skill, the first attempts are clumsy and slow, and show few results. It is easier to return to old ways than to continue trying to master new and sometimes difficult tasks. The best way to master new skills is through practice and evaluation of the results.

Self-Management Skills

What you do about something is largely determined by how you think about it. For example, if you think that having a chronic illness is like falling into a deep pit, you may have a hard time motivating yourself to crawl out, or you may even think the task is impossible. The thoughts you have can greatly determine what happens to you and how you handle your health problems.

Some of the most successful self-managers are people who think of their illness as a path. This path, like any path, goes up and down. Sometimes it is flat and

11

smooth. At other times the way is rough. To negotiate this path one has to use many strategies. Sometimes you can go fast, other times you must slow down. There are obstacles to negotiate.

Good self-managers are people who have learned the skills to negotiate this path. These skills fall into three main categories:

12

- *Skills needed to deal with the illness*
  Any illness requires that you do new things. These may include taking medicine, using an inhaler, or using oxygen. It means more frequent interactions with your doctor and the health care system. Sometimes there are new exercises or a new diet. All of these constitute the work you must do to just manage your illness.

- *Skills needed to continue your normal life*
  Just because you have a chronic illness does not mean that life does not go on. There are still chores to do, friendships to maintain, jobs to perform, and a multitude of family relationships that continue. Things that you once took for granted can become much more complicated in the face of chronic illness. You may need to learn new skills in order to maintain your daily activities and to enjoy life.

- *Skills needed to deal with emotions*
  When you are diagnosed as having a chronic illness, your future changes, and with this comes changes in plans and changes in emotions. Many of these emotions are negative. They may include anger: "Why me? It's not fair"; depression: "I can't do anything any more, what's the use"; frustration: "No matter what I do it doesn't make any difference. I can't do what I want to do"; or isolation: "No one understands, no one wants to be around someone who is sick." Negotiating the path of chronic illness, then, also means learning skills to work with these negative emotions.

Self-Management Tasks

1.   **To take care of your illness** (*such as taking medicine, exercising, going to the doctor, communicating your symptoms accurately, changing diet*).

2.   **To carry out your normal activities** (*chores, employment, social life, etc.*).

3.   **To manage your emotional changes** (*changes brought about by your illness, such as anger, uncertainty about the future, changed expectations and goals, and sometimes depression, and you can include changes in your relationship with family and friends*).

With this as background, you can think of self-management as the use of skills to

1. manage the work of dealing with your illness,
2. manage the work of continuing your daily activities, and
3. manage the changing emotions brought about by chronic illness.

Throughout this book you will find information to help you learn and practice self-management skills. This is *not* a textbook. You do not need to read every word in every chapter. Instead, read the first two chapters and then use the *table of contents* to find the information you need. Feel free to skip around. In this way you will learn the skills you need to negotiate your individual path.

• • •

Suggested Further Reading

Cousins, Norman. *Anatomy of an Illness as Perceived by the Patient: Reflections on Healing and Regeneration.* New York: W.W. Norton and Co., 1995.

Klein, Robert A., and Marcia Goodman Landau. *Healing: The Body Betrayed.* Minneapolis: DCI/CRONIMED Publishing, 1992. (Self-paced, self-help guide to regaining psychological control of your chronic illness.)

Moore, James E., Kate Long, Michael Von Korff, Virginia M. Gonzalez, and Diana D. Laurent. *The Back Pain Help Book.* Reading, Mass.: Perseus, 1999.

Register, Cheri. *Living With Chronic Illness: Days of Patience and Passion.* New York: Bantam Books, 1989.

Sobel, David, and Robert Ornstein. *Healthy Pleasures*, 2nd ed. Reading, Mass.: Addison-Wesley, 1997.

CHAPTER
2

Becoming an Active Self-Manager

IT IS IMPOSSIBLE TO HAVE A CHRONIC CONDITION WITHOUT BEING A SELF-MANAGER. Some people manage by withdrawing from life. They stay in bed or socialize less. The disease becomes the center of their existence. Other people with the same condition and symptoms somehow manage to get on with life. They may have to change some of the things they do or the way that things get done. Nevertheless, life continues to be full and active. The difference between these two extremes is not the disease but rather how the person with a chronic condition decides to manage the disease.

Like any skill, active self-management must be learned and practiced. This chapter will start you on your way. Remember: ***You are the manager.*** Like the manager of an organization or a household you must

1. *decide* what you want to accomplish,
2. look for *alternative ways* to accomplish this goal,
3. start making *short-term* plans by making an action plan or agreement with yourself,
4. *carry out* your action plans,
5. *check* the results,
6. make *changes* as needed, and
7. remember to *reward* yourself.

Problems sometimes start with a general uneasiness. Let's say you are unhappy but not sure why. Upon closer examination, you find you miss contact with some distant relatives. With the problem identified, you decide to take a trip to visit these relatives. You know what you *want to accomplish.*

In the past, you have always driven but find it tiring, so you seek *alternative ways* of travel. Among other things, you consider leaving at noon instead of early in the morning and making the trip in two days instead of one. You consider asking a friend along to share the driving. There is also a train that goes within 20 miles of your destination, or you might fly (although the airport is not very convenient). You decide to take the train.

The trip still seems overwhelming, as there is so much to do to prepare. You decide to write down all the steps necessary to make the trip a reality. These include finding a good time to go, buying a ticket, figuring out how to handle luggage, seeing if you can make it up and down the stairs to get on the train, wondering if you can walk on a moving train to get food or go to the bathroom, and figuring out how you will get to the station.

You start by *making an action plan* for yourself that this week you will call and find out just how much the railroad can help. You also decide to start taking a short walk each day and walking up and down a few steps so that you can be steadier on your feet. Having done this, you *carry out your action plan* by calling the railroad and starting your walking program.

A week later you *check the results*. Looking back at all the steps to be accomplished, you find that a single call answered many questions. The railroad is used to people who have mobility problems and has dealt with many of your concerns. However, you are still worried about walking. Even though you are walking better, you are still unsteady. You make a change in your plan by asking a physical therapist about this and he suggests using a cane. Although you hate it, you find that a cane gives you that extra security needed on a moving train.

Now you are ready to make a new action plan for accomplishing some of the other tasks necessary to make the trip possible. What once seemed like a dream is becoming a reality.

Now let's go through these seven steps in detail. They are the backbone of any self-management program.

Deciding What You Want to Accomplish

Deciding what you want to accomplish may be the most difficult part. You must be realistic and very specific.

Think of all the things you would like to do. One of our self-managers wanted to climb twenty steps to her daughter's home so that she could join her family for a holiday meal. Another wanted to lose weight to help his cardiac condition. Still another wanted to be more socially active but felt limited by the need to take her oxygen tank everywhere. In each case, the goal was one that would take several weeks or even months to accomplish.

In fact, one of the problems with goals is that they often seem like dreams. They are so far off that we don't even try to accomplish them. We'll tackle this problem next. For now, take a moment and write your goals here:

Goals:

1. _____

2. _____

3. _____

Put an asterisk (*) next to the goal you would like to work on first.

Looking for Alternative Ways of Accomplishing the Goal

Sometimes what keeps us from reaching our goal is a failure to see alternatives, or we reject alternatives without knowing much about them. In the earlier example, our traveler was able to make a list of alternate travel arrangements, and then chose the train.

There are many ways to reach any specific goal. For example, our self-manager who wanted to climb 20 steps could start off with a slow walking program, could start to climb a few steps each day, or could look into having the family gathering at a different place. The man who wanted to lose weight could decide not to eat between meals, to give up desserts, or to start an exercise program. The self-manager who wanted more social contact could find out about community college classes or Better Breathers clubs, or could call or write friends.

As you can see, there are many options for reaching each goal. The job here is to list the options and then choose one or two on which you would like to work.

Sometimes it is hard to think of all the options yourself. If you are having problems, it is time to use a consultant. Share your goal with family, friends, and health professionals. You can call community organizations such as the Heart or Lung Association or the Arthritis Foundation. You can use the Internet. Don't ask *what* you should do. Rather, ask for *suggestions*. It is always good to have a list of options.

Now a note of caution. Many options are never seriously considered because you assume they don't exist or are unworkable. Never make this assumption until you have thoroughly investigated the option. One woman we know had lived in the same town all her life and felt that she knew all about the community resources. When she was having problems with her health insurance, a friend from another city suggested contacting an insurance counselor. However, the woman dismissed this suggestion because she *knew* that this service did not exist in her town. It was only when, months later, the friend came to visit and called the area Agency on Aging (which exists in most counties in the U.S.) that the woman learned there were three insurance counseling services nearby. In short, never assume anything. Assumptions are major self-management enemies.

Write the list of options for your main goal here. Then put an asterisk (*) next to the two or three options on which you would like to work.

Options:

1. _____

2. _____

3. _____

4. _____

5. _____

6. _____

Making Short-Term Plans—Action Planning

The next step is to turn your options into *short-term plans*, which we will call an action plan. An action plan calls for a specific action or set of actions that you can realistically expect to *accomplish* within, say, the next week. The action plan should be about something **you** want to do or accomplish. This is a tool to help you do what **you** wish. You do not make action plans to please your friends, family, or doctor.

Action plans are probably your most important self-management tool. Most of us can do things to make us healthier, but fail to do them. For example, most people with chronic illness can walk, some just across the room, others for a half block. Most can walk several blocks, and some can walk a mile or more. However, few people have a systematic exercise program.

An action plan helps us to do the things we know we should do. Let us go through all the steps for making a realistic action plan. This is an important skill, which may well determine the success of your self-management program.

First, *decide what you will do this week.* For a step-climber this might be climbing three steps on four consecutive days. The man trying to lose weight may decide not to eat between meals for three days and to walk around the block before dinner on the following four days. This action must be something you want to do, that you feel you can do realistically, a step on the way to your long-term goal.

Make sure that your plans are "behavior specific"; that is, rather than just deciding "to relax," you will "listen to my progressive muscle relaxation tapes."

Next, *make a specific plan.* This is the most difficult and important part of making an action plan. Deciding what you want to do is worthless without a plan to do it. The plan should contain all of the following steps:

1. *Exactly **what** are you going to do?* How far will you walk, how will you eat less, what breathing technique will you practice?

2. ***How much** will you do?* Will you walk around the block, walk for 15 minutes, not eat between meals for three days, practice breathing exercises for 15 minutes?

3. ***When** will you do this?* Again, this must be specific, such as before lunch, in the shower, when I come home from work. Connecting a new activity with an old habit is a good way to make sure it gets done. Another trick is to do your new activity before an old favorite activity such as reading the paper or watching a favorite TV program.

4. ***How often** will you do the activity?* This is a bit tricky. We would all like to do things every day, but it is not always possible. It is usually best to decide to do something three or four times a week. If you do more, so much the better. However, if you are like most of us, you will feel less pressure if you can do your activity three or four times and still be successful at your action plan. (Please note! Taking medications is an exception. This must be done exactly as directed by your doctor.)

There are a couple of rules for writing your action plan that may help you achieve success. First, *start where you are* or start slowly. If you can walk only for one minute, start your walking program with walking one minute once every hour or two, not with walking a mile. If you have never done any exercise, start with a few minutes of warm-up. A total of five or ten minutes is enough. If you want to lose weight, set a goal based on your existing eating behaviors, such as not eating after dinner.

Also, *give yourself some time off.* All people have days when they don't feel like doing anything. That is a good reason for saying that you will do something three times a week instead of every day. That way, if you don't feel like walking one day, you can still achieve your action plan.

Once you've made your action plan, *ask yourself* the following question: "On a scale of 0 to 10, with 0 being totally unsure and 10 being totally confident, *how confident am I* that I can complete this plan?

If your answer is 7 or above, this is probably a realistic action plan. Congratulate yourself, you have done the hard work. If your answer is below 7, then you should look again at your action plan. Ask yourself why you're not confident. What problems do you foresee? Then see if you can either solve the problems or change your plan to make yourself more confident of success.

Once you have made a plan you are happy with, *write it down* and post it where you will see it every day. Keep track of how you are doing and the problems you encounter. (Page 24 is a completed example of an action plan. Page 25 is a blank copy; make copies of it to use weekly.)

Basics of a Successful Action Plan

1. Something YOU want to do

2. Reasonable *(something you can expect to be able to accomplish that week)*

3. Behavior-specific *(losing weight is **not** a behavior; not eating after dinner **is**)*

4. Answers the questions:

   What?

   How much?

   When? *(think about your day/week—which days, times, etc.?)*

   How often?

5. Confidence level of 7 or more *(that you will complete the **entire** contract)*

Carrying Out Your Action Plan

If the action plan is well written and realistic, fulfilling it is generally pretty easy. Ask family or friends to check with you on how you are doing. Having to report your progress is good motivation. Keep track of your daily activities while carrying out your plan. All good managers have lists of what they want to accomplish. Check things off as they are completed. This will give you guidance on how realistic your planning was and will also be useful in making future plans. Make daily notes, even of the things you don't understand at the time. Later these notes may be useful in establishing a pattern to use for problem solving.

For example, our stair-climbing friend never did her climbing. Each day she had a different problem: not enough time, being tired, the weather was too cold, and so on. When she looked back at her notes, she began to realize that the real problem was her fear of falling with no one around to help her. She then decided to use a cane while climbing stairs and to do it when a friend or neighbor was around.

Checking the Results

At the end of each week, see if you completed your action plan and if you are any nearer to accomplishing your goal. Are you able to walk farther? Have you lost weight? Are you less fatigued? Taking stock is important. You may not see progress day by day, but you should see a little progress each week. At the end of each week, check on how well you have fulfilled your action plan. If you are having problems, this is the time to problem solve.

Making Midcourse Changes (Problem Solving)

When trying to overcome obstacles, the first plan is not always the most workable plan. If something doesn't work, don't give up. Try something else; modify your short-term plans so that your steps are easier, give yourself more time to accomplish difficult tasks, choose new steps to your goal, or check with your consultants for advice and assistance.

The first and most important step in problem solving is to *identify the problem.* This is usually the most difficult step, as well. You may know, for example, that stairs are a problem for you, but it will take a little more effort to determine that the real problem is fear of falling.

Once you have identified the problem, the next step is to *list ideas to solve the problem.* You may be able to come up with a good list yourself, but often calling in help from consultants is helpful. Consultants can be friends, family, members of your health care team, or community resources.

When you have a list of ideas, *pick one to try.* As you try something new, remember that new activities are usually difficult. Be sure to give your potential solution a fair chance before deciding it won't work.

Assess the results after you've given your idea a fair trial. If all goes well, your problem will be solved.

If you still have the problem, *substitute another idea* from your list and try again.

If a solution still eludes you, *utilize other resources* (your consultants) for more ideas. If all of the above does not work, then you may have to *accept that your problem may not be solvable right now.* This is sometimes hard to do. Just because a problem is not solvable right now doesn't mean that it won't be solvable later or that other problems can't be solved in the same way. Even if your path is blocked, there are probably alternate paths. Don't give up. Keep going.

Summary of Problem-Solving Steps

1. Identify the problem *(this is the most difficult and most important step)*.
2. List ideas to solve the problem.
3. Select one method to try.
4. Assess the results.
5. Substitute another idea if the first didn't work.
6. Utilize other resources *(ask friends, family, professionals for ideas if your solutions didn't work)*.
7. Accept that the problem may not be solvable now.

Rewarding Yourself

The best part of being a good self-manager is the reward you will get in accomplishing your goals and living a fuller and more comfortable life. However, don't wait until your goal is reached, rather reward yourself frequently. For example, decide that you won't read the paper until after your exercise. Thus, reading the paper becomes your reward. One self-manager buys only one or two pieces of fruit at a time and walks the half-mile to the supermarket every day or two to get more fruit. Another self-manager who stopped smoking used the money he would have spent on cigarettes to have his house professionally cleaned, and there was even enough left over to go to a baseball game with a friend. Rewards don't have to be fancy, expensive, or fattening. There are many healthy pleasures that can add enjoyment to your life.

In review, a successful self-manager

1. sets goals,
2. makes a list of alternatives for reaching the goal,
3. makes short-term action plans toward that goal,

4. carries out the plan,
5. checks on progress weekly,
6. makes midcourse changes as necessary, and
7. uses rewards for a job well done.

One last note: Not all goals are achievable. Chronic illness may mean having to give up some options. If this is true for you, don't dwell too much on what you can't do. Rather, start working on another goal you would like to accomplish. One self-manager we know who uses a wheelchair talks about the 90% of the things he can do. He spends his life developing this 90% to the fullest.

Now that you understand the meaning of self-management, you are ready to begin using the tools that will make you a self-manager. Even if your particular illness or condition does not have a specific chapter, this book is still for you. The chart on pages 7–9 may contain information that will point you toward the specific self-management skills you'll need. Remember: Most self-management skills are similar for all diseases. Chapters 15 to 18 contain information on some of the more common chronic illnesses. In Chapter 14 we talk about medications and their uses. The rest of the book is devoted to tools of the trade. These include exercise, nutrition, symptom management, communication, making decisions about the future, finding resources and information about the durable power of attorney for health care, and, of course, sex and intimacy.

Action Plan Form

In writing your action plan, be sure it includes
1. what you are going to do,
2. how much you are going to do,
3. when you are going to do it, and
4. how many days a week you are going to do it.

For example: This week, I will walk (what) around the block (how much) before lunch (when) three times (how many).

This week I will _____ *walk around the block* _____ (what)

_____ *3 times* _____ (how much)

_____ *before lunch* _____ (when)

_____ *3 days this week* _____ (how many)

How confident are you? (0 = not at all confident; 10 = totally confident) __*9*__

	Check off	Comments
Monday	—	*raining*
Tuesday	✓	*walked slowly & noticed everything around me*
Wednesday	✓	*It was cool out, but the walk felt good*
Thursday	—	*raining again*
Friday	✓	*only walked around the block 2 times*
Saturday	✓	*took a friend along—we had a nice chat*
Sunday	—	*felt tired*

Action Plan Form

In writing your action plan, be sure it includes
1. what you are going to do,
2. how much you are going to do,
3. when you are going to do it, and
4. how many days a week you are going to do it.

For example: This week, I will walk (what) around the block (how much) before lunch (when) three times (how many).

This week I will_____(what)

_____(how much)

_____(when)

_____(how many)

25

How confident are you? (0 = not at all confident; 10 = totally confident)_____

	Check off	**Comments**
Monday		
Tuesday		
Wednesday		
Thursday		
Friday		
Saturday		
Sunday		

CHAPTER
3

Finding Resources

A MAJOR PART OF BECOMING A SELF-MANAGER OF YOUR CHRONIC ILLNESS is knowing when you need help and how to find help. Seeking help to perform daily tasks, to assist with chores, or to help with other areas of your life does *not* mean that you have fallen victim to your illness. Instead, knowing where to go for help in specific areas of your life takes initiative, evaluation of your condition and your own capabilities. By becoming more aware of the symptoms you experience throughout the day, you can better predict the amount of energy and patience you will have later to accomplish tasks. If you find that you come up short on energy, time, patience, or capability for some tasks, you can evaluate where help from other resources will spare you for those things most important to you.

The first resource we probably go to for help is *family,* followed by *close friends.* Some find it difficult, however, to ask for help from people they know. Finding the right words to ask for help is discussed in Chapter 10. Unfortunately, some people either do not have family or close friends to call on, or cannot bring themselves to ask. If this is the case, you must look for other resources in your community.

Finding resources in your community can be a little like a "treasure hunt." Just like a treasure hunt, creative thinking wins the game. Finding what you need may be as simple as looking in the telephone book and making a couple of phone calls. Other times, it may take detective talents to find it. The community resource detective must find clues and follow them, including starting over when the clue leads to a dead end.

Finding and recognizing clues are the detective's most important task. For example, suppose you find it difficult to prepare meals because prolonged standing is too tiring or painful. However, after some thought, you decide that you want to continue cooking for yourself rather than have someone else cook your meals.

So you must explore getting your kitchen altered to enable you to prepare meals from a seated position.

Where can you find an architect or contractor who has knowledge and experience in kitchen alterations for people with physical limitations? You need a starting point for your treasure hunt. Looking at the yellow pages and the classified section of the newspaper reveals pages of ads and listings for architects and contractors; some ads say they specialize in kitchens, but others don't mention any specialty. None mention anything about designing for physical limitations. A couple of phone calls to those listing kitchens as a specialty are unsuccessful in finding anyone experienced in kitchens for the physically limited.

Now what? Well, you have a couple of choices in your hunt for clues. First, you can call everyone listed until you find what you need. Not only would this be time-consuming, but you may not feel comfortable about the person you find until you talk to someone else who knows his work.

Who else do you know that might have information of this kind? Maybe someone who works with physically disabled people would know, such as an occupational or physical therapist, an orthopedic supply store, your city or county's human services department or commission, the nearest independent living center for the disabled, the community college disabled services office, or the local chapter of the Heart Association, the Lung Association, the Diabetes Association, or the Arthritis Foundation, for example.

You may talk to someone who doesn't have the answer but will say, "Gosh, Jack so-and-so just had his kitchen remodeled to accommodate his wheelchair. Maybe he can help you find someone." Jack's name is probably a great clue. He may be able not only to give you the name of someone who does the work, but also some ideas about cost and hassle before you go any further in the process. He's probably done much of the detective work already.

Suppose, however, that your search still isn't successful. There are people in every community who are natural community resources. These "Naturals" seem to know everyone and where everything is in their community. They tend to be folks who have lived a long time in the community and have been involved in it. They are natural problem-solvers.

You may already know such a person. The "Natural" is the one people always seek out for advice, and they always seem to be helpful. You probably count him or her among your friends or acquaintances. If you were to call this person, he or she would probably know the answer or set you on the right path to get the answer. Sometimes the "Natural" will taste the thrill of the hunt and, like a modern-day Sherlock Holmes, will announce that "the game is afoot!" and promptly join you in your search.

The "Natural" could be a friend, a business associate, the mail carrier, your physician, your pet's veterinarian, the checker at the corner grocery, the pharmacist, the bus or taxi driver, your kid's school secretary, a real estate agent, the Chamber of Commerce receptionist, or the librarian. All you need do is think of this person as an information resource.

Watch out, though! Once you get good at thinking about community resources creatively, you will become a "Natural" in your community!

Resources for Resources

When we need to find goods or services, there are certain resources we can call on in order to find more resources. The *"Natural"* is one of those resources, but our community resource "detective's kit" needs a variety of other tools to be fully useful.

Probably the most frequently used tool we pull from our community resource detective's kit is the *telephone book.* Particularly if you can hire someone to do something for you, the phone book is full of people and organizations ready to help. For most searches, this is where to start.

While you have your telephone book out, another tool to look up is your local *information and referral service* number. There are several types of agencies that operate these extremely helpful services. Look under the United Way Information and Referral, Senior Information and Referral (or Area Agency on Aging, Council on Aging), and "information and referral" in your county or city government listings. Once you have an information and referral telephone number, your searches will become much easier. These services maintain a huge file of referral addresses and telephone numbers for just about any help you might need. Even if they don't have the answer to your need, they will almost always be able to refer you to another agency who can speed you along in your search.

One of the most important resources you can find for either information or help is the *voluntary agencies* dedicated to your disease. In the United States, these include the American Heart Association (for stroke as well as heart disease), the American Lung Association, the American Diabetes Association, and the National Arthritis Foundation. There are similar organizations in most other countries. These agencies, funded by contributions from individuals and from corporate sponsors, provide up-to-date information about your disease, as well as support and direct services to people with the disease. They also fund research that they hope will help people live better with their disease and someday lead to a cure. For a small membership fee, you can become a member of these organizations, entitling you to receive regular bulletins by mail. You do not, however, have to be a member to qualify for their services. They are here to serve you. Many of these organizations have wonderful Web sites. In our new world of cyberspace, you can live in rural North Dakota and get help on the Web from the Arthritis Foundation in Victoria, Australia.

There are *other organizations* in your community offering information and referral services along with direct services. These include the local chapter of the American Association of Retired Persons (AARP), senior centers, community centers, and religious social service agencies. These organizations offer information, classes, recreational opportunities, nutrition programs, legal and tax help, and social programs. There is probably a senior center or community center close to you. Your city government office or local librarian will know where they are, and the calendar section of your newspaper will usually have information about programs these organizations offer.

Most *religious groups* offer information and social services to those who need it, either directly through the local church or synagogue or through the Council of Churches, Catholic Diocese, or Jewish social service groups. To get help from religious organizations, start with the local church or synagogue, and they will help you or refer you to someone who can help you. You need not be a member of the religion or of its local organization to receive help.

Your *hospital or health care organization* may also offer services. Call your local hospital, clinic, or health insurance plan and ask for their social service departments. Your doctor will also be aware of the services available in the health care organizations he or she is affiliated with.

The next resource to call upon in your search is the *library*. Particularly when you are looking for information about your disease, this is a valuable resource. The library, and the *reference librarian* in particular, can provide an information and referral service as well. Often the reference section of the library will have a little gem of a book or pamphlet that will give you listings of the resources you are looking for. If you're a good detective, you will find the gem on your own. The reference librarian, on the other hand, can probably take you right to it (and maybe show you some others, too). Even if you think you are an excellent detective in the library, it's a good idea to ask the reference librarian to see whether you have overlooked something. These people see volumes of material cross their desks, and are knowledgeable about the community (probably "Naturals" as well).

In addition to the city or county library we are most familiar with, there are other, more specialized libraries available to us. Ask your information and referral service if there is a "health library" in your community. These libraries specialize in health-related resources, sometimes even having a computerized database search service available, along with the usual print, audiotape, and videotape

30

materials. These libraries are usually offered through nonprofit organizations and hospitals, and will sometimes charge a small fee for use.

Universities and colleges also have libraries open to the public. By law, in fact, the regional *"government documents"* sections of these libraries must be open to the public at no charge. Government publications exist on just about any subject, and the health-related publications are particularly extensive. You can find information on everything from organic gardening to detailed nutritional recipes. The librarians are usually very helpful, and these publications are "your tax dollars at work."

If you are fortunate enough to have a medical school in your community, you may be able to use their *medical library.* This, however, is a place to go for information, rather than a place to look for help with tasks. Naturally, you would expect to find a great deal of information about disease and treatment at a medical library. Unless you have some special knowledge about medicine, however, the information you find in a medical library can be intimidating, confusing, and possibly frightening. Use medical libraries with care.

Many books related to your disease will have reading lists and resource lists at the backs of the books. Sometimes we miss the *"backs of books"* bibliographies because these lists are found around or after the index. "Backs of books" are helpful for either finding information or finding agencies or other organizations.

Your *local newspaper* is also an excellent resource, and the health editor, science editor, or the "calendar of events" editor can be very knowledgeable about resources in the community. The two sections of the newspaper that can be most helpful in your search for resources are the *"calendar of events"* section and the *"classified"* section. Organizations advertise classes, lectures, and other events in these sections. Even if you are not interested in the particular event advertised, the contact telephone number given may be an important clue in your search for something else. Look in other logical places for news stories that might be of interest also, such as the pages around the calendar section or the sports and fitness section (if you are looking for an exercise program for people with your health problem, for example).

Sometimes you can find clues in the classified section, as well. Look under "announcements," "health," or any other heading that seems promising. Review the index of classified headings that is usually printed at the front of the classified section near the rate information to see which headings your newspaper uses.

Information Overload—The Internet

The fastest growing resource in our society today is the Internet. Information is being added to this worldwide network at a dizzying rate every day, every second.

The Internet (all electronic information transfer, including e-mail and graphical Web pages) and the World Wide Web (the graphical interface to the Internet that we are most familiar with) not only offer nearly endless supplies of information about health and anything else you can imagine, but also opportunities to interact with other people all over the world. Someone who has a rare health condition might find it difficult to find others with the same disease to talk to near where she or he lives. With the Internet, though, there might be a whole group of people to talk to—it doesn't matter whether they are across the street or on the other side of the world.

The good thing about the Internet is that anyone can have a Web site. The bad thing about the Internet is that anyone can have a Web site. The Internet has virtually no controls about who is posting information or whether the information is correct, or even safe. This can mean that there is a lot of information out there that might be very useful, because individuals can share information quickly. It can also mean that someone might post incorrect or dangerous information, as well. No one should ever assume that information seen on the Internet is true. Approach the information with skepticism and caution: Is the author/sponsor of the Web site clearly identified? Is the author reputable? Is the information contrary to what everyone else seems to say about the subject? Does common sense support the information? What is the purpose of the Web site? Are they trying to sell you something?

One quick way to start analyzing the purpose of the Web site is to look at the URL (the address, starting with http://). The URL usually will look something like this:

http://www.stanford.edu/

"http://" begins every Web URL. It means "hyper text transfer protocol." "www" means that the server (computer) that Stanford University's main Web site lives on is dedicated to the World Wide Web. "stanford" identifies that the server belongs to Stanford University. "edu" indicates that Stanford University is an education institution.

Looking at the last part of the main part of a Web site's URL, you will most often see .edu, .org, .gov, or .com if they originate in the United States. This will give you a clue about the nature of the organization that owns the Web site. A college or university will have .edu, a nonprofit organization will have .org, a governmental agency will have .gov, and a commercial organization will have .com. As a *general* rule of thumb, .edu, .org, and .gov will be pretty trustworthy sites, although a nomprofit organization can be formed to promote just about anything. A Web site with .com is trying to sell you a product or service, or they are selling advertising space on their site to others trying to sell you something. This doesn't mean that a commercial Web site can't be a good one. On the contrary, there are many outstanding commercial Web sites dedicated to giving us good-quality, trustworthy information. They are often able to do this service only by selling advertising or by accepting grants from commercial firms. (They have to pay their bills, too!) Here are some of our favorite URLs that can get you started. The "links" pages on these sites are like "backs of books." "Links" are URLs that will send you to that Web site simply by clicking on it.

National Institutes of Health:
    http://www.nih.gov/
Centers for Disease Prevention and Control:
    http://www.cdc.gov/
Office of Rare Diseases, NIH:
    http://cancernet.nci.nih.gov/ord/info-diseases.html
U.S. Department of Health and Human Services:
    http://www.healthfinder.gov/
Tufts University Nutrition Navigator:
    http://navigator.tufts.edu/
Johns Hopkins University Health Information:
    http://www.intelihealth.com/IH/ihtIH
University of Washington HealthLinks:
    http://www.hslib.washington.edu/
Ask NOAH:
    http://www.noah.cuny.edu/
Mayo Clinic:
    http://www.mayohealth.org/
Former Surgeon General Dr. Koop's site:
    http://www.drkoop.com/
Dr. Dean Edell's site:
    http://www.healthcentral.com/
Health AtoZ:
    http://www.healthatoz.com/
Health News Directory:
    http://www.healthnewsdirectory.com/HealthNews/Directory/
The Patients Guide to Healthcare Information on the Internet:
    http://www3.bc.sympatico.ca/me/patientsguide/
Pharmaceutical Information Network:
    http://pharminfo.com/drugdb/db_mnu.htm.
RxList—the Internet Drug Index:
    http://www.rxlist.com/

Becoming an effective community resource detective is one of the jobs of a good self-manager. Hopefully, this chapter has given you some ideas about the process of finding resources in your community. Knowing how to search for resources will serve you better than being handed lists of resource agencies. To get you started in your search, we have included at the end of each appropriate chapter a "Community Resource Detective's Kit" like the one below.

Community Resource Detective's Kit

Finding Resources

The "Natural"

The Telephone Book

Information and Referral Service

Voluntary Agencies

Senior Center, Community Center, Religious Organization

Hospital, Health Care Organization

The Library and Reference Librarian

The Internet

"Backs of Books"

CHAPTER
4

Understanding Common Symptoms

CHRONIC ILLNESSES COME WITH SYMPTOMS. These symptoms are signals from the body that something unusual is happening. They cannot be seen by others, are often difficult to describe to others, and are usually unpredictable. While some symptoms are common, when they occur, and the way in which they affect us, is very personal. These symptoms, which include fatigue, stress, shortness of breath, pain, itching, anger, depression, and sleep problems, can interact with each other; this in turn can worsen existing symptoms and/or lead to new symptoms or problems.

Regardless of the causes of these symptoms, the ways in which we can manage them are similar. This chapter discusses some of the symptoms most common among different conditions, as well as some of their causes. In addition, some ways to deal with the symptoms are discussed. In Chapter 5, cognitive techniques are discussed; these are the ways you can use your mind to help deal with these symptoms.

Dealing With Common Symptoms

Learning to manage symptoms is very similar to the process of problem solving that was discussed in Chapter 2 (page 21). Before you can manage a symptom, it is important to identify which symptom you are experiencing. Next, it is necessary to try to determine the cause of the symptom at this particular time. While this may sound like a simple process, it is not always easy because symptoms and the problems caused by chronic disease can be numerous, complex, and often interrelated.

The person with a chronic condition can experience many different symptoms, and each symptom can have various causes. The way in which these symptoms

Tips for Practicing Different Symptom-Management Techniques

- **Choose a technique to try first.** Be sure to give this method a fair trial. We recommend that you practice it twice a day for at least two weeks before deciding whether or not the technique is going to be helpful to you.

- **Try some other techniques, giving each the same trial period.** It is important to try more than one technique because some may be more useful for some symptoms, or you may find that you simply prefer some techniques over others.

- **Think about how and when you will use each technique you have chosen.** For example, some of these methods may require more substantial lifestyle changes. As you practice the different techniques, you may find that some work best for specific symptoms and not so well for others. The best symptom managers learn to use a variety of techniques according to their needs and situation on a daily basis.

- **Place some cues in your environment to remind you to practice these techniques as both practice and consistency are important for the mastery of new skills.** For example, place stickers or notes where you'll see them, such as on your mirror, near the phone, in your office, or on the car's dashboard. Also, change the notes periodically so that you'll continue to notice them.

- **Try linking the practice of each technique with some other established behavior or activity in your daily routine.** For example, practice relaxation as part of your cool-down from exercise. Also, ask a friend or family member to remind you to practice each day; he or she may even wish to participate.

affect one's life is also different. All of these factors can become very tangled like the loose threads of a cloth. To be able to successfully manage these symptoms, we must figure out how to untangle the threads.

As you read through this chapter, you will note that many symptoms have the same causes. Also, one symptom may actually cause other symptoms. By gaining a better understanding of the possible causes of your symptoms, you will be better able to identify more effective ways to deal with these symptoms and their causes. As you learn more about the causes, you may also find ways to prevent certain symptoms from recurring.

Now let's look at some of the more common symptoms experienced by people with different chronic conditions.

Fatigue

Having a chronic condition can drain your energy. Therefore, fatigue is a very real problem for many people. It is *not*, as some might say, "all in the mind." Fatigue can keep you from doing things you'd like to do. Often, it is misunderstood by those who do not have a chronic illness. Unfortunately, spouses, family members, and friends sometimes do not understand the unpredictable way in which the fatigue associated with your condition can affect you. They may think that you are just not interested in certain activities or that you want to be alone. Sometimes you may not even know why you feel this way.

To be able to manage fatigue, it is important to understand that your fatigue may be related to several factors, such as

- *The disease itself.* Whether the disease is diabetes, emphysema, chronic bronchitis, asthma, or heart or liver disease, activities demand more energy. When a chronic illness is present, the body is less efficient in its use of the energy reserved for everyday activities, in part, because some of this energy is used to help the body heal itself.

- *Inactivity.* Muscles that are not used become deconditioned and less efficient in doing what they are supposed to do. The heart, which is made of muscular tissue, can also become deconditioned. When this happens, the ability of the heart to pump blood, necessary nutrients, and oxygen to other parts of the body is decreased. When muscles do not receive these necessary nutrients and oxygen, they cannot function properly. Deconditioned muscles tire more easily than muscles in good condition—those that receive an adequate supply of blood, oxygen, and nutrients.

- *Poor nutrition.* Food is our basic source of energy. If the fuel we take in is not good quality and/or in the proper quantities, fatigue can result. For some people, obesity results in fatigue. Extra weight causes an increase in the amount of energy needed to perform daily activities. For others, being underweight can cause problems associated with fatigue. This is especially true for those with chronic obstructive pulmonary disease (COPD). Many people with COPD experience sudden weight loss because of a change in their eating habits and therefore have increased fatigue.

- *Insufficient rest.* For a variety of reasons, there are times when we do not get enough sleep or have poor quality sleep. This can also result in fatigue. Later in this chapter, sleep problems will be discussed in more detail.

- *Emotions.* Stress and depression can also cause significant fatigue. Most people are aware of the connection between stress and feeling tired, but fewer are aware of the fact that fatigue is a major symptom of depression.

If fatigue is a problem for you, your first job is to *determine the cause.* Are you eating healthy foods? Are you exercising? Are you getting enough good quality sleep? If you answer "no" to any of these questions, you may be well on your way to determining one or more of the reasons for your fatigue.

The important thing to remember about your fatigue is that it may be caused by things other than your illness. Therefore, in order to combat and prevent fatigue, you must address the different causes of your fatigue. This may mean trying a variety of techniques.

If your fatigue is caused by *not eating well,* such as eating too many "empty calories" in the form of "junk food" or alcohol, then the solution is to eat better quality foods in the proper quantities. For others, the problem may be a decreased interest in food, leading to a lack of calories and subsequent weight loss. Chapter 13 discusses, in greater detail, some of the problems associated with eating, as well as tips for improving your eating habits.

People often say they can't exercise because they feel fatigued. Believing this creates a vicious cycle: People are fatigued because of a *lack of exercise,* and yet, they don't exercise because of the fatigue. Believe it or not, if this is your problem, then motivating yourself to do a little exercise the next time you are fatigued might be the answer. You don't have to run a marathon. The important thing is to get outdoors and take a short walk. If this is not possible, then walk around your house. See Chapter 6 for more information on getting started on an exercise program.

If *emotions* are causing your fatigue, rest will probably not help. In fact, it may make you feel worse, especially if your *fatigue is a sign of depression.* We will talk about how to deal with depression a little later in this chapter. If you feel that your fatigue may be related to stress, then read the next section for some tips on managing stress.

Stress

Stress is a common problem for everyone. But what **IS** stress? In the 1950s, physiologist Hans Selye described stress as "the nonspecific response of the body to any demand made upon it." Others have expanded this definition to explain that the body adapts to demands, whether pleasant or unpleasant.

How Does Your Body Respond to Stress?

Your body is used to functioning at a certain level. When there is a need to change this level, your body must adjust physiologically to meet the demand. Your body reacts by preparing itself to take an action: Your heart rate increases, your blood pressure rises, your neck and shoulder muscles tense, your breathing becomes more rapid, your digestion slows, your mouth becomes dry, and you may begin sweating. These are signals of "stress."

- *Why does this happen?* To take an action, your muscles need to be supplied with oxygen and energy. Your rate of breathing increases in an effort to inhale as much oxygen as possible and to get rid of as much carbon dioxide as possible. Your heart rate increases to deliver the oxygen and nutrients to the muscles. Furthermore, physiological processes that are not immediately necessary, such as the digestion of food and the body's natural immune responses, are slowed down.

- *How long will these responses last?* In general, these responses are present only until the stressful event passes. Then your body returns to its normal level of functioning. Sometimes, though, your body does not return to its former comfortable level. If the stress is present for any length of time, your body begins adapting to this stress. This adaptation can contribute to other problems such as hypertension, shortness of breath, or muscle and joint pain.

Common Types of Stressors

Regardless of the type of stressor, the changes in the body are the same. Stressors, however, are not completely independent of one another. In fact, one stressor can often lead to other types of stressors or even magnify the effects of existing stressors. Several stressors can also occur simultaneously. This is much the same as the "vicious cycle" described in Chapter 1. Let us look now at some of the more common sources and types of stress.

- *Physical stressors.* The physical stressors can range from something as pleasant as picking up your grandchild for the first time, to grocery shopping, to the physical symptoms of your chronic illness. The one thing these three stressors have in common is that they all increase your body's demand for energy. If your body is not prepared to deal with this demand, the results may range from sore muscles to fatigue to a worsening of some disease symptoms.

- *Mental and emotional stressors.* The mental and emotional stressors can range from pleasant to uncomfortable. The joys you experience from seeing a child get married or meeting new friends induce the same stress response in the body as feeling frustrated or down because of your illness. While it seems strange that this is true, the difference comes in the way the stress is perceived by your brain.

- *Environmental stressors.* The environmental stressors can also be both good and bad. These stressors may be as varied as a sunny day, uneven sidewalks that make it difficult to walk, loud noises, bad weather, or secondhand smoke.

Isn't "Good Stress" a Contradiction?

As we mentioned earlier, some types of stress can be good, such as a job promotion, a wedding, a vacation, a new friendship, or a new baby. These stressors make you feel good, but still cause the physiological changes in your body that were discussed above. Another example of a "good stressor" is exercise.

When you exercise, or do any type of physical activity, there is a demand placed on the body. The heart has to work harder to deliver blood to the muscles; the lungs are working harder and you breathe more rapidly to keep up with your muscles' demand for oxygen. Meanwhile, your muscles are working hard to keep up with the signals from your brain which are telling them to keep moving.

As you maintain an exercise program for several weeks, you will begin to notice a change: What once seemed virtually impossible is now relatively simple. Your body has adapted to this stress. In addition, there is less strain on your heart, lungs, and other muscles to do this extra work. They've become more efficient, and you have become more fit.

Recognizing When You Feel Stressed

Everyone has a certain need for stress. It helps your life run more efficiently. As long as you do not go past the "breaking point," stress is helpful. Some days you can tolerate more stress than on others. But sometimes, if you are not aware of the different types of stress you are experiencing, you can go beyond this breaking point and feel like your life is completely out of control. Often it is difficult to recognize when you are under too much stress. Some warning signs include

- biting your nails, pulling your hair, or other repetitive habits,
- grinding your teeth, clenching your jaw,
- tension in your head, neck, or shoulders,
- feelings of anxiousness, nervousness, helplessness, irritability, and
- frequent accidents or forgetting things you usually don't forget.

41

Sometimes, you can catch yourself when you are behaving or feeling these ways. If you do, take a few minutes to think about what it is that is making you feel tense. Take a few deep breaths and try to relax. (Some relaxation methods are presented in Chapter 5.)

Let us now examine how to deal with stress.

Dealing with Stress

Avoiding Stressful Situations

There are some situations that you recognize as stressful, such as being stuck in traffic, going on a trip, or preparing a meal. First, *look, as objectively as possible, at what it is about the particular situation that is stressful.* Is it that you hate to be late? Are trips stressful because of the uncertainty involved with your destination? Does meal preparation involve too many steps that demand too much energy?

Once you have decided on the problem, *begin looking for possible ways to reduce the stress.* Can you leave earlier? Can you let someone else drive? Can you call someone at your destination site and ask about wheelchair access, local mass transit, and so on? Can you prepare food in the morning? Can you take a short nap in the early afternoon?

After you have identified some possible solutions, *select one* to try the next time you are in this situation. Don't forget to *evaluate the results.* (This is the problem-solving approach that was discussed in Chapter 2.)

Managing the Stress

While you can successfully manage some types of stress by modifying the situation, other types of stress seem to sneak up on you when you don't expect them. The approach to dealing with this type of stress also involves problem solving.

If you know that certain situations will be stressful, *develop ways to deal with them before they happen.* Try to *rehearse,* in your mind, what you will do when the situation arises so that you will be ready. Inherent in this approach is the ability to listen to and recognize your body's signals that the tension and stress are building. The better you become at listening and understanding your body signals, the better you'll become at managing your stress and stressful situations.

Certain chemicals you may consume can also increase stress. These chemicals include nicotine, alcohol, and caffeine. Although some people tend to smoke a cigarette, drink a glass of wine, or drink a cup of coffee to soothe their tension, this, in fact, actually increases the body's stress response. Eliminating or cutting down these stressors can leave you feeling calmer.

The cognitive techniques discussed in the next chapter may also be useful to you during stressful situations; these are self-talk, progressive muscle relaxation, guided imagery, and visualization.

Some additional ways to deal with stress include getting enough sleep, exercising, and eating well. These are also discussed in other chapters of this book.

In summary, stress, like every other symptom, has many causes and therefore can be managed in many different ways. It is up to you to examine the problem and try those solutions that meet your needs and lifestyle.

Shortness of Breath

Shortness of breath, like fatigue and stress, can be related to several factors. In all cases, your body is not getting the oxygen it needs. The difference comes in the types of physiological changes that take place as the result of a chronic illness. These changes can lead to an increased sensitivity to different stimuli. (Before reading further about shortness of breath, you may wish to turn first to Chapter 15, which discusses normal lung functioning, as well as changes that take place in the lungs with chronic lung disease.) Some of the most common changes that can take place are discussed below.

Damage to the air sacs in the lungs, as is the case with emphysema, causes the lungs to be less efficient at getting oxygen into the blood and carbon dioxide out. While the body can adjust to this change to some extent, when there is a sudden change in the "normal" breathing pattern, the lungs cannot always keep up.

Narrowing of the airways to the air sacs and *excess mucus production* are associated with chronic bronchitis. Because the airways become narrowed, there is less room for air to flow through to get to the lungs. Therefore, your body receives less oxygen.

42

People with *asthma* have problems similar to those of chronic bronchitis. One difference between these two diseases is that with asthma, the narrowing of the airways, coupled with an increase in mucus production, is in response to some sort of stimulus.

People with *heart disease* can also experience problems with shortness of breath, but for different reasons. With heart disease, the heart becomes *less efficient* at pumping blood throughout the body. If there is a sudden change in the demand for oxygen by the body, the heart has to work harder to deliver this oxygen. Because the heart cannot work hard enough to meet the oxygen needs of the body, a person can feel short of breath, as the breathing rate speeds up to try to meet this need. This increase in the breathing rate can make a person feel even more short of breath.

People who are *overweight* can experience shortness of breath because the added weight increases the amount of energy, and therefore oxygen, required by the body to do even simple tasks. This also increases the workload for the heart. If obesity is coupled with chronic lung disease or heart disease, there is added difficulty in supplying the body with the oxygen it needs.

Deconditioning of muscles can also lead to shortness of breath. This deconditioning process can affect the breathing muscles or any of the other muscles in your body. When muscles become deconditioned, they are less efficient in doing what they are supposed to do, so they require more energy (and oxygen) to perform activities than do well-conditioned muscles. In the case of the breathing muscles, the problem is complicated by muscle deconditioning because clearing the lungs becomes less efficient. This leaves less space for fresh air to be inhaled.

Just as there are many causes of shortness of breath, there are many things you can do to manage this problem.

When you feel short of breath, *don't stop what you are doing or hurry up to finish, but slow down.* If shortness of breath continues, then stop for a few minutes. If you are still short of breath, take your medication, if it has been prescribed by your doctor. Often, shortness of breath is frightening and this fear can cause two additional problems. First, the hormones that fear itself can release may cause more shortness of breath. Second, fear may cause you to stop your activity and thus never build up the endurance necessary to help your breathing. The basic rule is to take things slowly and in steps.

Increase your activity level gradually, generally not by more than 25% each week. Thus, if you are now able to garden comfortably for 20 minutes, next week, increase it by a maximum of five minutes. Once you can garden comfortably for 25 minutes, you can again add a few more minutes.

Don't smoke, and equally important, *avoid smokers.* This may sometimes be difficult, because smoking friends may not realize how difficult they are making your life. Your job is to tell them. Explain that their smoke is causing breathing

43

problems for you and that you would appreciate it if they would not smoke when you are around. Also, make your house and especially your car "No Smoking" zones. Ask people to smoke outside.

Use your medications and oxygen as prescribed by your doctor. We are constantly being bombarded by messages that drugs are bad and not to be used. In many cases, this is correct. However, when you have a chronic disease, drugs can be, and often are, life savers.

Don't try to skimp, cut down, or go without. Likewise, more is not better, so don't take more than the prescribed amount of medication(s), either. Drugs, taken as prescribed, can make all the difference. This may mean using medications even when you are not having symptoms. This also means resisting the temptation to take more of the medication if the prescribed amount does not seem to be working. If you have questions about your medications or feel they are not working for you, discuss these concerns with your doctor *before* you stop taking the medication or take more than has been prescribed. Preventing problems before they start is much better than having to manage the problem.

Drink plenty of fluids if mucus and secretions are a problem, unless your doctor has advised you to restrict your fluid intake. This will help to thin the mucus and, therefore, make it easier to cough up. The use of a humidifier may also be helpful.

Practice *pursed-lip and diaphragmatic breathing.* As mentioned earlier, one of the problems that causes shortness of breath, especially for people with emphysema, chronic bronchitis, and asthma, is a deconditioning of the diaphragm and breathing muscles. When this deconditioning occurs, the lungs are not able to empty properly, leaving less room for fresh air.

Practiced together, pursed-lip and diaphragmatic breathing can help strengthen and improve the coordination and the efficiency of the breathing muscles, as well as decrease the amount of energy needed to breathe. In addition, these two exercises can be used with any of the cognitive symptom-management techniques that use the power of your mind to manage your symptoms (described in Chapter 5) or alone, to achieve a state of relaxation.

The following are the steps for *pursed-lip breathing.* You can use this technique during exercise or any time you feel short of breath.

1. *Breathe in through your nose.* (This may be easier if you lean forward.)
2. *Hold your breath* briefly.
3. *With your lips pursed* (as if you were going to whistle), *breathe out slowly* through your lips. Exhaling should take **twice** as long as inhaling.

4. *Practice* this technique for five to ten minutes, two to four times a day.

Diaphragmatic breathing requires a little more practice to master than pursed-lip breathing. While pursed-lip breathing helps to empty the lungs of trapped air and reestablish a normal breathing pattern, diaphragmatic breathing strengthens the breathing muscles. Strengthening these muscles makes them more efficient, so less effort is needed to breathe. The following are the steps for diaphragmatic breathing:

1. *Lie on your back* with pillows under your head and knees.
2. Place *one hand on your stomach* (at the base of your breastbone) and the *other* hand on your upper chest.
3. *Inhale slowly through your nose,* allowing your stomach to expand outward. Imagine that your lungs are filling with fresh air. The hand on your stomach should move upward, and the hand on your chest should not move or move only slightly.
4. *Breathe out slowly, through pursed lips.* At the same time, use your hand to gently push inward and upward on your abdomen.
5. *Practice* this technique for ten to fifteen minutes, three or four times a day, until it becomes automatic. If you begin to feel a little dizzy, rest.

45

Once you feel comfortable doing this, you may wish to place a light weight on your abdomen. This will help to further strengthen the muscles used to inhale. Start with a weight of about one pound, like a book or a bag of rice or beans. Gradually increase the weight as your muscle strength improves. After you can breathe easily lying down, you can practice diaphragmatic breathing while sitting, standing, and finally, while walking. By mastering this technique while doing other activities, you will be better able to manage your shortness of breath.[1]

Pain/Physical Discomfort

Pain or physical discomfort is a problem shared by many people with chronic illness. In fact, for many people, this is their number one concern. As with most symptoms of chronic illness, this pain or discomfort can have many causes. The four most common causes are

---

[1] The material on pursed-lip and abdominal, or diaphragmatic, breathing was taken from the following two publications: *Essentials of Pulmonary Rehabilitation* by Thomas L. Petty, M.D., Brian Tiep, M.D., and Mary Burns, R.N., B.S. Pulmonary Education and Research Foundation, P.O. Box 1133, Lomita, CA 90717-5133; and *Help Yourself to Better Breathing,* American Lung Association, 1989.

- *The disease itself.* Pain can come from inflammation, damage in or around joints and tissues, insufficient blood supply to the heart, or trapped nerves, to name just a few.
- *Tense muscles.* When something hurts, the muscles in that area become tense. This is your body's natural reaction to *pain*—to try to protect the damaged area. When muscles are tensed for a period of time, lactic acid builds up in the muscles which can also cause soreness or pain.
- *Muscle deconditioning.* With chronic disease, it is common to become less active, leading to a weakening of the muscles, or muscle deconditioning. When a muscle is weak, it tends to complain any time it is used. This is why even the slightest activity can sometimes lead to pain and stiffness.
- *Lack of sleep or poor quality sleep.* Pain often interferes with the ability to get either enough sleep or good quality sleep. This, in turn, can make pain worse, as well as lessen your ability to cope with it.
- *Stress, anxiety, and emotions such as depression, anger, fear, and frustration.* These are all normal responses to living with a chronic condition, and they can affect your perception of the pain or discomfort. When we are stressed, angry, afraid, or depressed, everything, including the pain, seems worse.

Because the pain comes from many sources, the methods we use to manage or reduce this pain must be aimed at all of these that apply. The use of medications can help with some of the disease pain. For example, medications can help open blood vessels and bronchial tubes. Other medications may reduce pain caused by inflammation.

With chronic disease, painkillers, such as narcotics, are generally *not* useful. Furthermore, narcotics can be dangerous for people with impaired respiratory function, because these drugs slow down the breathing rate, making existing breathing problems worse. Painkillers also tend to be less effective over time and are usually addictive. Since chronic disease is long-term and the associated pain can also be long-term, the potential for addiction to high doses of painkillers is greatly increased.

Two of the best ways to deal with pain are the use of exercise and cognitive symptom-management techniques, such as relaxation and visualization, in which you actively use your mind to help reduce your symptoms. The benefits of exercise as well as tips for starting an exercise program are discussed in Chapters 6 through 9. Using your mind to manage symptoms is discussed in Chapter 5.

In addition to exercise and the use of cognitive techniques, there are several other methods that are sometimes useful for localized pain. These include the use of *heat, cold, and massage*. These three applications work by stimulating the skin and other tissues surrounding the painful area, which, in turn, increases the blood flow to these areas.

Stimulation with *heat* can be done by applying a heating pad or by taking a warm bath or shower (with the water flow directed at the painful area).You can make a heating "pad" by placing rice or dry beans in a sock, knotting the top of the sock, and placing it in a microwave oven for three to four minutes. Before use, be sure to test the heat so as not to burn yourself. Some people, however, prefer *cold* for soothing pain, especially if there is inflammation. A bag of frozen peas or corn makes an inexpensive, reusable cold pack. Whether using heat or cold, limit the application to 15 or 20 minutes at a time.

Massage is one of the oldest forms of pain management. Hippocrates (c. 460–380 B.C.) said "physicians must be experienced in many things, but assuredly also in the rubbing that can bind a joint that is loose and loosen a joint that is too hard." Self-massage is a simple procedure that can be performed with little practice or preparation. It stimulates the skin, underlying tissues, and muscles with applied pressure. Some people like to use a mentholated cream with self-massage because it also gives a cooling effect.

Massage, while relatively simple, is not appropriate for all cases of pain. Do *not* use self-massage for a "hot joint" (one that is red, swollen, and hot to the touch) or an infected area or if you are suffering from phlebitis, thrombophlebitis, or skin eruptions.

If pain continues to have a major influence on your life, you might ask for a referral to a pain-management clinic.

Itching

Of all the symptoms one may have, itching is one of the most difficult to understand and even harder to define. Basically, itching is any sensation that causes an urge to scratch. Itching, like other symptoms, can have many different causes. Some of these we understand such as the itching caused by the release of histamines that irritate nerve endings. This happens when you get an insect bite or come in contact with some substance such as poison ivy or oak. People with liver diseases may also experience itching that is caused by the deposit of bile products in the skin when the liver is damaged and cannot function properly to remove them. There is, however, no association between the amount of bile products deposited and the amount of itching that one may experience. In kidney disease, itching may be severe but the exact cause is not clear. There are also other conditions, such as psoriasis, where the causes of itching are not easily explained. We do know that other factors such as warmth, wool clothing, and stress can make itching worse. The following are some ways that may help you relieve your itching.

Moisture

48

Dry skin tends to be itchy; therefore, it is important to keep the skin moisturized by applying moisturizing creams several times a day. When you choose a moisturizer, be careful. Just because a product is advertised as a moisturizer does not necessarily mean it is. Be sure to read the list of ingredients when buying a cream or lotion. Avoid products that contain alcohol or any other ingredient that ends in "ol," which is usually some variation of alcohol. These types of ingredients actually tend to dry the skin, rather than moisturize it. In general, the greasier the product, the better it works as a moisturizer. Creams are better moisturizers than lotions, and products such as Vaseline or vegetable shortening are also very effective.

When taking a bath or shower, use warm water and soak for not less than 10 or more than 20 minutes. You also may want to add bath oil, baking soda, or "Sulzberger's household bath oil" to the water. This household bath oil is made from 2 teaspoons of olive oil and a large glass of milk, which is added to the bath. When you get out of the water, pat yourself dry immediately and apply your cream.

If your itching is caused by the release of histamines during an allergic reaction or from having had contact with an irritating substance, it is important to wash off the oils or offending agent, apply cold compresses, and take Benadryl to help block the histamines.

During cold weather it can be especially difficult to deal with the itching because the indoor heating tends to dry the skin. If this is a problem for you, the use of a humidifier might help. Also, try to keep your home and office as cool as you can without being uncomfortable.

Clothing

The type of clothing you wear can also add to the itching sensations; therefore, it is important to select the appropriate clothing. Obviously, the best rule of thumb is to wear what is comfortable. This is usually clothing made from material that is not scratchy. Most people find that natural fibers such as cotton allow the skin to "breathe" better and are the least irritating on the skin.

Medications

Antihistamines will help if your itching is caused by the release of histamines. You can buy many of these products over the counter. They include triprolidine (Actifed), diphenhydramine (Benadryl), and chlorpheniramine maleate (Chlor-Trimeton).

You can also buy creams that help to soothe the nerve endings such as Ben Gay and Vicks VapoRub. If you want an anti-itch cream, look for ones that contain benzocaine, lidocaine, or pramoxine. However, be careful because some people can have allergic reactions to these creams, especially benzocaine. Capsaicin creams may also help itching, although they will cause a burning sensation. Steroid creams can also help control some types of itching. These are creams that contain cortisone or other steroids.

If you are confused about what over-the-counter products to buy, ask your doctor or pharmacist.

With the exception of moisturing creams, none of the other types of creams should be used on a long-term basis without talking to your doctor. If your itching continues with use of these over-the-counter products, you may want to talk to your doctor about trying the strong prescription versions of these medications.

Stress

Anything that you can do to reduce the stress in your life will also help reduce the itching. We have already discussed some of the ways to deal with stress earlier in this chapter, and there are some other techniques described in Chapter 5 (Using Your Mind to Manage Symptoms).

Scratching

While our natural tendency is to scratch what itches, this really does not help, especially for chronic itching. Rather, it leads to a vicious cycle whereby the more you scratch, the more you tend to itch. Unfortunately, it is hard to resist scratching. However, you might try rubbing, pressing, or patting the skin when you feel the need to scratch. If you are not able to break this cycle yourself, consult with a dermatologist who may be able to help you find alternative ways to control the itching.

Itching is a common and, undoubtedly, a very frustrating symptom for both patients and physicians to manage. When the self-management tips described here do not seem to help, it may be time to utilize the help of a physician. Often, he or she can offer some prescription medications that can help with some specific types of itching. Also, if you are interested in learning more about itching, we recommend the book written for physicians titled *Itch Mechanisms and Management of Pruritus* by Jeffrey D. Bernard (McGraw-Hill, 1994). You might also recommend this book to your doctor.

Anger—"Why Me?"

50

Anger is one of the most common responses to chronic illness. The uncertainty and unpredictability of living with a chronic disease threatens what you have fought all your life to achieve—independence and control. The loss of control over your body and loss of independence in life create feelings of frustration, helplessness, and hopelessness, all of which fuel the anger. In fact, at various times during the course of your illness, you may find yourself asking, "Why me?" You may wonder what you did to deserve this or why God is punishing you. All of these are normal anger responses to chronic disease.

You may be angry with yourself, family, friends, health care providers, God, or the world in general—all for a variety of reasons. For example, you may be angry at yourself for not taking better care of yourself when you were younger. You may be angry at your family and friends because they don't do things the way you would like them done. Or you might be angry at your doctor because he or she cannot "fix" your problems. Sometimes your anger may be misplaced, as when you find yourself yelling at the cat or dog. Misplaced anger is quite common, especially if you are not even aware that you are angry or why.

Sometimes, the anger is not just a response to having a chronic illness, but is actually the result of the disease process itself. For example, if someone has suffered a stroke that affected a certain part of the brain, that person's ability to express or suppress emotions may be affected. Thus, some people who have had strokes may appear to cry inappropriately or have flares in temper.

Recognizing (or admitting) that you are angry and identifying why, or with whom, are important steps to learning how to manage your anger effectively. This task also involves finding constructive ways to express your anger. If not expressed, the anger becomes unhealthy. It can build up until it becomes explosive and offends others, or is turned inward, thereby intensifying the experience of other disease symptoms like depression.

There are several things that you can do to help manage your anger. One important way is to learn how to *communicate your anger verbally,* preferably without blaming or offending others. This can be done by learning to use "I" (rather than "you") messages to express your feelings. (Refer to Chapter 10 for a discussion of "I" messages.) However, if you choose to express your anger verbally, know that many people will not be able to help you. Most of us are not very good at, or comfortable, dealing with angry people, even if the anger is justified. Therefore, you may also find it useful to seek counseling or join a support group. Voluntary organizations, such as the Heart, Lung, Liver, and Diabetes Associations and the Arthritis Foundation, may be useful resources in this area.

Another way to deal with anger is to *modify your expectations*. You have done this throughout your life. For example, as a child you thought you could become anything, a fireman, a ballet dancer, a doctor, etc. As you grew older, however, you reevaluated these expectations, along with your capabilities, talents, and interests. Based on this reevaluation, you modified your plans.

This same process can be used to deal with the effects of chronic illness on your life. For example, it may be unrealistic to expect that you will get "all better." However, it is realistic to expect that you can still do many pleasurable things. You have the ability to affect the progress of your illness, by slowing its decline or preventing it from becoming worse. Changing your expectations can help you to change your perspective. Instead of dwelling on the 10% of things you can no longer do, think about the 90% of things you still can do. You may even be able to find new activities or hobbies to replace those old ones. Developing a more positive attitude and positive self-talk can also help to change your perspective; this is discussed more in the next chapter.

Anger can also be *channeled through new activities,* such as exercise, writing, music, or painting. Some people find these extremely therapeutic outlets for this emotion.

In short, *anger is a normal response to having a chronic condition.* Part of learning to manage the condition involves acknowledging this anger and finding constructive ways to deal with it.

Depression

Depression can be a scary word. Some people prefer saying that they are "sad," "blue," or "feeling down." Whatever you call it, depression is a normal reaction to chronic illness.

Sometimes it is not easy to recognize when you are depressed. Even more difficult is recognizing when you may be becoming depressed and then catching yourself before you fall into a deep depression. Just as there are many degrees of pain, there are different degrees of depression. If your disease is a significant problem in your life, you almost certainly have or have had some problems with depression. Depression is felt by everyone at some time. It is how you handle it that makes the difference.

51

While there are many signs of depression, which will be discussed later in this section, there are also several emotions that can lead to depression. These include the following:

- *Fear, anxiety, and/or uncertainty about the future.* Whether these feelings result from worries about finances, the disease process, or your family, constant worry about these issues can lead to depression if they are not addressed by you and those involved. Chapter 19 deals with some decisions all of us will have to make at some time in our lives. By confronting these issues early on, both you and your family will need less time to worry about them and have more time to enjoy life.

- *Frustration can have any number of causes.* You may find yourself thinking, "I just can't do what I want," "I feel so helpless," "I used to be able to do this myself," or "Why doesn't anyone understand me?" Feelings like these can leave you feeling more alone and isolated the longer you hold on to them.

- *Loss of control over your life.* Whether it comes from having to rely on medications to ease symptoms, having to see a doctor on a regular basis, having to count on others to help you perform daily activities such as bathing, dressing, and preparing meals, this feeling of losing control can make you lose faith in yourself and your abilities. Your life has suddenly become a team sport in which you are no longer the coach. Instead, you are now a player with someone *else* calling the plays.

While these feelings have been described separately, they are often experienced in combination, making it more difficult to determine what is really at the root of the depression. Also, we often do not recognize when we are depressed, or do not wish to admit to ourselves that we are actually depressed.

The following are 13 common signs of depression. Learning to recognize the signs of depression is the first step in learning how to manage it.

1. *Loss of interest in friends or activities.* Not wanting to talk to anyone or to answer the phone or doorbell. In short, isolation is an important symptom of depression.
2. *Difficulty sleeping,* changed sleeping patterns, interrupted sleep, or sleeping more than usual. Often, going to sleep easily but awakening and being unable to return to sleep occurs.
3. *Changes in eating habits.* This change may range from a loss of interest in food to unusually erratic or excessive eating.

4. *Unintentional weight change,* either gain or loss, of more than 10 pounds in a short period of time. (This can also be a sign of physical illness and should be checked out by your doctor.)
5. *Loss of interest in personal care and grooming.*
6. *A general feeling of unhappiness* lasting longer than six weeks.
7. *Loss of interest in being held or in sex.* Sometimes these problems can also be due to medication side effects, so it is important that you talk them over with your doctor.
8. *Suicidal thoughts.* If your unhappiness has caused you to think about killing yourself, get some help from your doctor, good friends, a member of the clergy, a psychologist, or a social worker. These feelings will pass and you will feel better, so get help and don't let a tragedy happen to you and your loved ones.
9. *Frequent accidents.* Watch for a pattern of increased carelessness, accidents while walking or driving, dropping things, and so forth. Of course you must take into account the physical problems caused by your disease such as unsteady balance or slowed reaction times which could also account for some accidents.
10. *Low self-image.* A feeling of worthlessness, a negative image of your body, wondering if it is all worth it.
11. *Frequent arguments or increased irritability.* A tendency to blow up easily over minor matters, over things that never bothered you before.
12. *Loss of energy.* Fatigue. Feeling tired all the time.
13. *Inability to make decisions.* Feeling confused and unable to concentrate.

53

Not all depression behavior is negative. Sometimes *unrealistic "cheeriness"* will mask what the person is really feeling, and the wise observer will recognize the brittleness or "phoniness" of the mood. *Refusal to accept offers* of help, even in the face of obvious need for it, is a frequent symptom of unrecognized depression.

Depression behavior tends to be excessive in one direction or another from what would be considered normal for that individual.

The paradox of depression-related behavior is that the more one engages in the behavior, the more likely it is that one will ultimately drive away the people who are most able to provide the comfort and support that the depressed person needs. Most of our friends and family want to help us feel better, but often they don't really know what to do to help. As their efforts to comfort and reassure us are frustrated, they may at some point throw up their hands and quit trying. Then the depressed person winds up saying "see, nobody cares," thus reinforcing the feelings of loss and loneliness.

Some of these signs of depression may seem familiar to you. Whether you've experienced these feelings in the past or are currently experiencing one or more of them, depression is a very real and common symptom associated with chronic illness.

Having a chronic illness, alone, can be very depressing. Although this is not a matter of how you should or should not feel, being depressed is not pleasant, and depression is something that can be managed. In fact, there are at least a dozen things you can do to change the situation. But if you are depressed, you may not feel like making the effort to do so. Force yourself or get someone to help you into action. Find someone to talk with.

Here are 13 things you can do:

1. *If you feel like hurting yourself or someone else,* call your mental health center, doctor, suicide prevention center, a friend, spiritual counselor, or senior center. **Do not delay. Do it now.** Often, just talking with an understanding person or health professional will be enough to help you through this mood.

2. *Are you taking tranquilizers or narcotic painkillers* such as Valium, Librium, reserpine, codeine, Vicodin, sleeping medications, or other "downers"? These drugs intensify depression, and the sooner you can stop taking them, the better off you will be. Your depression may be a drug side effect. If you are not sure what you are taking or are uncertain if what you're experiencing could be a side effect, check with a doctor or pharmacist. Before discontinuing a prescription medication, *always* check, at least by phone, with the prescribing physician, as there may be important reasons for continuing its use or there may be withdrawal reactions.

3. *Are you drinking alcohol* in order to feel better? Alcohol is also a downer. There is virtually no way to escape depression unless you unload your brain from these negative influences. For most people, one or two drinks in the evening is not a problem, but if your mind is not free of alcohol during most of the day, you are having trouble with this drug. Talk this over with your doctor or call Alcoholics Anonymous.

4. *Continue your daily activities.* Get dressed every day, make your bed, get out of the house, go shopping, walk your dog. Plan and cook meals. Force yourself to do these things even if you don't feel like it.

5. *Visit with friends,* call them on the phone, plan to go to the movies or on other outings. Do it!

54

6. *Join a group.* Get involved in a church group, a discussion group at a senior center, a community college class, a self-help class, or a senior nutrition program.

7. *Volunteer.* People who help other people are seldom depressed.

8. *Make plans and carry them out.* Look to the future. Plant some young trees. Look forward to your grandchildren's graduation from college even if your own kids are in high school. If you know that one time of the year is especially difficult, such as Christmas or a birthday, make specific plans for that period. Don't wait to see what happens. Be prepared.

9. *Don't move to a new setting* without first visiting for a few weeks and learning about the resources available to you in this new community. Moving can be a sign of withdrawal, and depression often intensifies when you are in a location away from friends and acquaintances. Besides, many types of troubles usually move with you, whereas the support you may need to deal with them effectively does not.

10. *Take a vacation* with relatives or friends. Vacations can be as simple as a few days in a nearby city or a resort just a few miles down the road. Rather than go alone, look into trips sponsored by colleges, city recreation departments, the "Y," senior centers, or church groups. Many people have found that Elder Hostel programs offer a vacation, as well as an opportunity to expand your knowledge of an interesting topic and to make new friends.

11. *Do 20 to 30 minutes of physical activity or exercise every day.*

12. *Make a list of self-rewards.* Take care of yourself. You can reward yourself by reading at a set time, seeing a special play, or with anything, big or small, that you can look forward to during the day.

13. *Use positive self-talk.* This cognitive technique is a very powerful weapon against depression. See Chapter 5 for more information on self-talk.

Depression feeds on depression, so *break the cycle*. The success of your self-management program depends on it. Depression is not permanent, and you can hasten its disappearance. Focus on your pride, your friends, your future goals, and your positive surroundings. How you respond to depression can be a self-fulfilling prophecy. When you believe that things will get better, they will.

Sleep Problems

Sleep is a time during which the body can concentrate on healing, because minimal amounts of energy are required to maintain body functioning when we sleep. When we do not get enough sleep, we can experience a variety of other symptoms, such as fatigue and a lack of concentration. But this does not mean that fatigue or lack of concentration are always caused by a lack of sleep. Remember, the symptoms associated with chronic disease can have many causes. If you have noticed a change in your sleep patterns, then the fatigue you are experiencing may be, at least in part, related to your problems with sleep. Some tricks to help you get a good night's sleep include:

Before you even get into bed

- *Get a comfortable bed* that allows for ease of movement and good body support. This usually means a good quality, firm mattress that supports the spine and does not allow the body to stay in the middle of the bed. A bed board, made of half-inch to three-quarter-inch (1 or 2 cm) plywood, can be placed between the mattress and the box spring to increase the firmness.
- Heated waterbeds or airbeds are helpful for some people with arthritis, because they support weight evenly by conforming to the body's shape. Other people can find them very uncomfortable. If you are interested, try one out at a friend's home or a hotel for a few nights to decide if it is right for you. An electric blanket or mattress pad, set on low heat, or a wool mattress pad are other effective ways of providing heat while sleeping, especially on cool or damp nights. If you decide to use electric bedding, be sure to follow the instructions carefully.
- *Find yourself a comfortable sleeping position.* The best position depends on you and your condition. Sometimes the use of small pillows placed in the right places can relieve pain and discomfort. Experiment with different positions and the use of pillows. Also, check with your health care provider for specific recommendations given your condition.
- *Elevate the head of the bed* on wooden blocks of four to six inches to make breathing easier. This same effect can be accomplished by use of pillows that elevate the chest, shoulders, and head.
- *Keep the room at a comfortable, warm temperature.*

- *Use a vaporizer* if you live where the air is dry. Warm, moist air often makes breathing easier, leaving you with one less thing to worry about when trying to fall asleep.
- *Make your bedroom a place in which you feel safe and comfortable.* Keep a lamp and telephone by your bed, easy to reach.
- If you are nearsighted and wear glasses or contact lenses, *keep a pair of glasses by the bed* when you go to sleep. This way, in case you need to get up in the middle of the night, you can easily put on your glasses and see where you are going!

Things to avoid before bedtime

- *Avoid eating before bedtime.* While you may feel sleepy after eating a big meal, this is no way to help you fall asleep and get a good night's sleep. Sleep is supposed to allow your body time to rest and recover, so when you eat, this takes valuable time away from this healing process. Since going to sleep feeling hungry may also keep you awake, try drinking a glass of warm milk at bedtime.
- *Avoid alcohol.* Contrary to the popular belief that alcohol will help you to sleep better because it makes you feel more relaxed, alcohol actually disrupts your sleep cycle. Alcohol, before bedtime, can lead to shallow and fragmented sleep, as well as frequent awakenings throughout the night.
- *Avoid caffeine late in the day.* Caffeine is a stimulant, and it can keep you awake. This includes coffee, some types of teas, colas, other sodas, and chocolate.
- *Avoid eating foods with MSG* (monosodium glutamate) late in the day. Although Chinese foods often have been singled out as containing MSG, many other types of food, especially pre-packaged foods, may contain this food additive. Before purchasing a pre-packaged meal, be sure to read the ingredient label to make sure it does not contain monosodium glutamate.
- *Don't smoke to help you sleep.* Aside from the fact that smoking itself can cause complications and a worsening of your chronic disease, falling asleep with a lit cigarette can be a fire hazard. Additionally, the nicotine contained in cigarettes is a stimulant.
- *Avoid diet pills.* Diet pills often contain stimulants, which may interfere with falling asleep as well as staying asleep.
- *Avoid sleeping pills.* While the name "sleeping pills" sounds like the perfect solution for sleep problems, they tend to become less

57

effective over time. Also, many sleeping pills have a rebound effect—that is, if you stop taking them, it is more difficult to get to sleep. Thus, as they become less effective, you have even more problems than you had when you first started taking the sleeping pills. All in all, it is best to avoid using sleeping pills if at all possible.

- If you are taking diuretics (water pills), you may want to take them in the morning so that your sleep is not interrupted so often by the need to go to the bathroom. Unless your doctor has recommended otherwise, don't reduce the overall amount of fluids you drink, as these are important for your health. However, you may want to limit your fluid intake right before you go to bed.

Develop a routine

- *Set up and maintain a regular rest and sleep schedule.* That is, go to bed at the same time every night and get up at the same time every morning. If you wish to take a nap, take one in the afternoon, but do not take a nap after dinner. Stay awake until you are ready to go to bed.
- If your sleep schedule is way off the norm (for example, you go to bed at 4 A.M. and sleep until noon), *reset your sleep clock.* To do so, try going to bed one hour earlier or later each day until you reach the hour you want to go to bed. This may seem strange, but it seems to be the best way to reset your sleep clock.
- *Exercise at regular times each day.* Not only will the exercise help you obtain a better quality sleep, it will also help to set a regular pattern during your day. However, avoid exercising immediately before bedtime, as well as other activities that excite you.
- *Get out in the sun every afternoon,* even if it is only for 15 or 20 minutes.
- Get used to doing the *same things every night before going to bed.* This can be anything from watching the news, to reading a chapter of a book, to taking a warm bath. By developing and sticking to a "time-to-get-ready-for-bed" routine, you will be telling your body that it's time to start winding down and relax.

"But I can't fall (back) asleep"

- *Only use your bed and your bedroom for sleeping.* If you find that you get into bed and you can't fall asleep, get out of bed and go into another room until you begin to feel sleepy again.

- Many people can get to sleep without a problem but then wake up and have the *"early morning worries"* where they can't turn off their minds. Then they get more worried because they cannot go back to sleep once they have awakened. Keeping your mind fully occupied will ward off the worries and help you get back to sleep. For example, try a distraction technique such as quieting your mind by counting backward from 100 by 3's or by naming a flower for every letter of the alphabet. The other relaxation techniques described in the next chapter may also be helpful.
- *Don't worry about not getting enough sleep.* If your body needs sleep, you will sleep. Also, remember that people tend to need less sleep as they get older.

Do you sleep "like a baby"?

If you fall asleep as soon as your "head hits the pillow," fall asleep regularly in front of the TV, and are tired when you wake up in the morning even after a full night's sleep, you may have a sleep disorder. People who have the most common sleep disorder, obstructive sleep apnea, often do not know it. When they are asked about their sleep, they respond "I sleep just fine." Sleep specialists believe that obstructive sleep apnea is very common and alarmingly underdiagnosed.

With sleep apnea, the soft tissue in the throat or nose relaxes during sleep and blocks the airway, causing extreme effort to breathe. The person struggles against the blockage for up to a minute, then wakes just long enough to gasp air, falling back to sleep to start the cycle all over again. The person is never aware that he or she has awakened dozens of times during the night and does not get the deep sleep needed to restore the body's energy and help with the healing process. This, in turn, leads to more symptoms such as fatigue and pain.

Sleep apnea is a serious medical problem and can be life-threatening. It has been linked to heart disease and stroke and is believed to be a cause of death for many who die in their sleep from a heart attack. Sleep experts suggest that people who are tired all the time in spite of a full night's sleep, or who find they need more sleep now than when they were younger, should be evaluated for sleep apnea or other sleep disorders, especially if they (or their spouses) report snoring.

In this section, we have discussed some common causes for some of the more common symptoms experienced by people with different chronic conditions. In addition, we have described some actions that you can take to cope with your symptoms. Taking action to physically deal with your symptoms is necessary in coping with your illness on a day-to-day basis. But sometimes, this just doesn't seem to be enough. There are times during the day during which you may wish to escape from your surroundings and just have "your time"—a time that allows you to clear your mind, to gain a fresh perspective. The following chapter presents different ways to complement your physical-symptom management with cognitive techniques, or using the power of your mind, to help reduce and even prevent some of the symptoms you may experience.

60

• • •

Suggested Further Reading

Ball, Nigel, and Nick Hough. *The Sleep Solution: A 21-Night Program for Restful Sleep.* Berkeley, Calif.: Ulysses Press, 1998.

Bernard, Jeffrey D. *Itch Mechanisms and Management of Pruritus.* New York: McGraw-Hill, 1994.

Billig, Nathan. *To Be Old and Sad—Understanding Depression in the Elderly.* Lexington, Mass.: D.C. Heath & Co., 1987.

Burton, Goldberg. *Alternative Medicine Guide to Chronic Fatigue, Fibromyalgia and Environmental Illness.* Tiburon, Calif.: Future Medicine Publishing, 1998.

Carter, Les, and Frank Minirth. *The Anger Workbook: A 13-Step Interactive Plan.* Nashville, Tenn.: Thomas Nelson, 1993.

Catalano, Ellen M., and Kimeron N. Hardin. *The Chronic Pain Control Work Book: A Step-By-Step Guide to Coping With and Overcoming Pain.* Berkeley, Calif.: New Harbinger, 1996.

Caudill, Margaret A. *Managing Pain Before It Manages You.* New York: Guilford Press, 1995.

Cooper, Kenneth H. *Can Stress Help? Converting a Major Health Hazard into a Surprising Benefit.* Nashville, Tenn.: Thomas Nelson, 1997.

Cunningham, J. Barton, and Bart Cunningham. *The Stress Management Sourcebook: Everything You Need To Know.* Chicago: Contemporary Publishing, 1997.

Falten, Sharon, and D. Diamond. *Tension Turnaround: The 30-Day Program for Inner Calm, Confidence and Control.* Emmaus, Pa.: Rodale Press, 1990.

Johnson, T. Scott, and Jerry Halberstadt. *Phantom of the Night.* Cambridge, Mass.: New Technology Publishing, 1995.

Kabat-Zinn, Jon, and Tich Nhat Hahn. *Full Catastrophe Living: Using the Wisdom of Your Body and Mind to Face Stress, Pain and Illness.* New York: Dell Publishing Co., 1991.

Kleinke, Chris L. *Coping With Life Challenges.* 2nd ed. Pacific Grove, Calif.: Brooks/Cole, 1997.

Lewinsohn, Peter, with Ricardo Munoz, Mary Youngren, and Antoinette Zeiss. *Control Your Depression.* New York: Simon and Schuster, 1992.

Natelson, Benjamin H. *Facing and Fighting Fatigue: A Practical Approach.* New Haven, Conn.: Yale University Press, 1998.

Powell, Trevor. *Free Yourself From Harmful Stress.* Chesham, England: Dorley Kindersley Ltd., 1997.

Schafer, Walt. *Stress Management for Wellness.* Fort Worth, Tex.: Harcourt Brace Jovanovich, 1995.

Seidman, David. *The Longevity Source Book.* Los Angeles: Lowell House, 1997.

Zammit, Gary. *Good Nights: How to Stop Sleep Deprivation, Overcome Insomnia and Get the Sleep You Need.* Kansas City, Mo.: Andrew McMeel Publishing, 1997.

61

CHAPTER
5

Using Your Mind to Manage Symptoms

ALL OF US, AT ONE TIME OR ANOTHER, HAVE EXPERIENCED THE POWER OF the mind and its effect on the body. Our thoughts and feelings, both pleasant and unpleasant, can cause the body to react in different ways. Oftentimes our heart rate and breathing are affected; we may experience other sensations such as perspiration, warm or cold, blushing, tears, and so on. Sometimes just a memory or an image can create these physiological responses. For example, take a moment now and think about a big, juicy lemon. Now begin to suck on the lemon. What happens? The body responds. Your mouth puckers and starts to water. You may even smell the scent of the lemon. All of these reactions are triggered by the mind and its memory of a lemon.

These examples demonstrate the power of the mind over the body and why we should develop our mental abilities to help us manage the different symptoms experienced by people with chronic conditions. Through training and practice, we can learn to use the mind to relax the body, to reduce stress and anxiety, and to reduce the discomfort or unpleasantness caused by physical and emotional symptoms. The mind can also effectively help to relieve the pain and shortness of breath associated with different diseases, and may even help a person depend less on the medications used to relieve some symptoms.

In this chapter we describe several ways in which you can begin to use your mind to manage symptoms. These are usually referred to as *cognitive techniques* because they involve the use of our thinking abilities to make changes in the body.

Relaxation Techniques

Many of us have heard and read about relaxation, yet some of us are still confused as to what relaxation is, its benefits, and how to do it. Relaxation is not a cure-all, but can be an effective part of a treatment plan.

There are different types of relaxation techniques, each having specific guidelines and uses. Some techniques are used only to achieve muscle relaxation, while others are aimed at reducing anxiety and emotional arousal, or diverting attention, all of which aid in symptom management.

The term "relaxation" means different things to different people. We can all identify ways we relax. For example, we may walk, watch TV, listen to music, knit, or garden. These methods, however, are different from the techniques discussed in this chapter because they include some form of physical activity that requires your mind's attention. Relaxation techniques are also different from taking a nap because we are using the mind actively to help the body achieve a relaxed state.

The goal of relaxation is to turn off the outside world so the mind and body are at rest. This allows you to reduce the tension that can increase the intensity or severity of symptoms.

Below are some guidelines to help you practice the cognitive techniques described in this chapter:

- *Pick a quiet place and time* during the day when you will not be disturbed for at least 15–20 minutes. (If this seems too long, start with 5 minutes.)
- Try to *practice the technique twice daily* and not less than four times a week.
- *Don't expect miracles.* Some of these techniques take time in order to acquire the skill. Sometimes it takes 3–4 weeks of consistent practice before you really start to notice benefits.
- *Relaxation should be helpful.* At worst, you may find it boring, but if it is an unpleasant experience or makes you more nervous or anxious, then you might try one of the other symptom-management techniques described in this chapter.

Muscle Relaxation

Muscle relaxation is one of the most commonly used cognitive techniques for symptom management. It is popular because it makes sense to us. If we are told that physical stress or muscular tension intensifies our pain, shortness of breath, or emotional distress, we are motivated to learn how to recognize this tension and release it.

In addition, muscle relaxation is easy to learn and remember for practice in different situations. It is also one technique from which we can recognize some immediate results, such as the positive sensations of reduced pain, stress, or muscle tension and calm, normal breathing. Muscle relaxation is not likely to fail because of distractions caused by symptoms or thoughts. It is a useful strategy to reduce pain, muscular tension, and stress, while helping to control shortness of breath and to achieve a more restful sleep.

The following are three examples of muscle relaxation techniques. Try each technique and choose the one that works best for you. Then you might want to tape record the script for that routine. Although this is not necessary, it is sometimes helpful if you find it hard to concentrate. Also, you won't be distracted by having to refer to the book when you are trying to relax.

Jacobson's Progressive Relaxation

Many years ago, a physiologist named Edmund Jacobson discovered that in order to relax, one must first know how it feels to be tense. He believed that if one learned to recognize tension, then one could learn to let it go and relax. He designed a simple exercise to assist with this learning process.

To relax muscles, you need to know how to scan your body, recognize where you are holding tension, and release that tension. The first step is to become familiar with the difference between the feeling of tension and the feeling of relaxation. This brief exercise will allow you to compare those feelings and, with practice, spot and release tension anywhere in your body. Pause for about 10 seconds whenever there is a series of dots (. . .).

Progressive Muscle Relaxation

Make yourself as comfortable as possible. Loosen any clothing that feels tight. Uncross your legs and ankles. Allow your body to feel supported by the surface on which you are sitting or lying.

Close your eyes. Take a deep breath, filling your chest and breathing all the way down to the abdomen. Hold . . . Breathe out through pursed lips, and, as you breathe out, let as much tension as possible flow out with your breath. Let all your muscles feel heavy and let your whole body just sink into the surface beneath you . . . Good.

This exercise guides you through the major muscle groups, asking you to first tense and then relax those muscles. If you have pain in a particular area today, tense those muscles only gently or not at all and focus on relaxing them.

Become aware of the muscles in your feet and calves. Pull your toes back up toward your knees. Notice the tension in your feet and calves. Release and relax. Notice the discomfort leaving as relief and warmth replace it. That's it.

Now tighten the muscles of your thighs and buttocks. Hold and feel the tension. Let go and allow the muscles to relax. The relaxed muscles feel heavy and supported by the surface upon which you are sitting or lying.

Tense the muscles in your abdomen and chest. Notice a tendency to hold your breath as you tense. Relax, and notice that it is natural to want to take a deep breath to relieve the tension in this area. Take a deep breath now, breathing all the way down to the abdomen. As you breathe out, allow all the tension to flow out with your breath.

Now, stretching your fingers out straight, tense your fingers and tighten your arm muscles. Relax. Feel the tension flowing out as the circulation returns.

Press your shoulder blades together, tightening the muscles in your shoulders and neck. This is a place where many people carry a lot of tension. Hold . . . Now, let go. Notice how the muscles feel warmer and more alive.

Tighten all the muscles of your face and head. Notice the tension, especially around your eyes and in your jaw. Now relax, allowing your jaw to become slack and your mouth to remain slightly open . . . That's right. Note the difference.

Now take another deep breath, breathing all the way down to the abdomen. And, as you breathe out, allow your body to sink heavily into the surface beneath you, becoming even more deeply relaxed. Good.

Enjoy this comfortable feeling of relaxation . . . Remember it. With practice, you will become skilled at recognizing muscle tension and releasing it . . .

Prepare to come back into the here and now. Take three deep breaths. And, when you're ready, open your eyes.

As Jacobson emphasizes, the purpose of voluntarily tensing the muscles is to learn to recognize and locate tension in your body. You will then become aware of tension and use this same procedure for letting it go. *Once you learn the technique, it will no longer be necessary to tense voluntarily; just locate the existing tension and let it go.*

For some people with a lot of pain, especially pain in the joints, the Jacobson technique may not be appropriate. If it causes any pain, this may distract from the relaxation. If this happens, try a different technique.

Body Scan

67

This is another relaxation technique, similar to Jacobson's progressive muscle relaxation exercise, but it does not require the tensing or movement of muscle groups. Like Jacobson, it is best done lying down on your back, but any comfortable position can be used. First, you must focus on your breathing. Spend a few minutes concentrating on each breath as it enters and leaves your body. Try directing your breath past your chest all the way down to your abdomen. (This is diaphragmatic breathing, which is described in Chapter 4 and is an important part of all relaxation exercises.)

> *After three or four minutes of concentrating on your breathing, move your attention to your toes. Don't move these, just think about how they feel. Don't worry if you don't feel anything at all. If you find any tension there, let it go as you breathe out.*
>
> *After a few moments of concentrating on your toes, move your attention to the bottoms of your feet. Again, don't move, just concentrate on any sensations you have. Let go of any tension you may find as you breathe out. Next concentrate on the top of your feet and your ankles. After a few more moments, bring your attention to your lower legs.*
>
> *Continue this process, shifting your attention every few moments to another part of your body, working slowly upward to your head. If you find tension, let it go as you breathe out. If your mind starts to wander, just bring your attention back to the feelings in your body and your breathing.*
>
> *This technique can also be used to help you get to sleep because it helps to clear your mind of any worries or distracting thoughts. The key is to give your full attention to scanning your body for tension and releasing it.*

The Relaxation Response

In the early 1970s, Dr. Herbert Benson studied extensively what he calls the "relaxation response." According to Dr. Benson, our bodies have several natural states. One example is the "fight or flight" response experienced by people when faced with a great danger. The body becomes quite tense, which is then followed by the body's natural tendency to relax; this is the relaxation response. As our lives become more and more hectic, our bodies tend to stay in an extended or constant state of tension, and we lose our ability to relax. In order to help our bodies relieve this tension and elicit the relaxation response, we may consciously need to practice the following exercise, which consists of four basic elements:

1. *A quiet environment* where there are few or no distractions.

2. *Find a comfortable position.* You should be comfortable enough to remain in the same position for 20 minutes.

3. *Choose a word, object, or pleasant feeling to dwell upon.* For example, repeat a word or sound like the word "one," gaze at a symbol like a flower, or concentrate on a feeling, such as peace.

4. *Adopt a passive attitude.* This is the most essential element. Empty all thoughts and distractions from your mind. You may become aware of thoughts, images, and feelings, but don't concentrate on them. Just allow them to pass on.

To elicit the relaxation response:

1. *Sit quietly* in a comfortable position.

2. *Close your eyes.*

3. *Relax all your muscles*, beginning at your feet and progressing up to your face. Keep them relaxed.

4. *Breathe in through your nose.* Become aware of your breathing. As you breathe out through your mouth, *say the word you chose* silently to yourself. Try to *empty all thoughts* from your mind; concentrate on your word.

5. *Continue* this for 10–20 minutes. You may open your eyes to check the time, but do not use an alarm. When you finish, sit quietly for several minutes, at first with your eyes closed. Do not stand up for a few minutes.

6. Do not worry about whether you are successful in achieving a deep level of relaxation. *Maintain a passive attitude* and let

relaxation occur at its own pace. When distracting thoughts occur, ignore them by not dwelling upon them, and return to repeating the word you chose.

7. *Practice* this once or twice daily, but ideally not within two hours after any meal. Digestive processes can interfere with relaxation responses.

This exercise is very much like meditation, which provides the principles on which the relaxation response is based. Meditation is discussed more later in this chapter.

69

While relaxation is the most common method for relieving muscle tension, other techniques can be used as supplements to provide additional emotional and/or cognitive benefits. These benefits include a reduction in fear and anxiety and a refocusing of attention away from the discomfort or unpleasantness of symptoms. These techniques include guided imagery and visualization.

Imagery

Guided Imagery

The guided-imagery relaxation technique is like a guided daydream. It allows you to divert your attention, refocusing your mind away from your symptoms and transporting you to another time and place. It has the added benefit of helping you to achieve deep relaxation by picturing yourself in a peaceful environment.

The guided imagery script presented here can help take you on this mental stroll. Again, consider each of the following ways to use imagery:

1. Read the script over several times to familiarize yourself with it. Then sit or lie down in a quiet place and try to reconstruct the scene in your mind. The script should take 15–20 minutes to complete.
2. Have a family member or friend read you the script slowly, pausing for about 10 seconds wherever there is a series of dots (. . .).
3. Make a tape of the script and play it to yourself whenever convenient.

Guided Imagery
Script

A Walk in the Country

Make yourself as comfortable as possible, sitting or lying down. Loosen any constricting clothing. Uncross your arms, legs, and ankles. Allow your body to feel supported by the surface on which you are sitting or lying.

Close your eyes.

Take a deep breath, in through your nose, breathing all the way down to the abdomen. Hold . . . Breathe out slowly through slightly pursed lips, and, as you do, relax your whole body, allowing all your muscles to feel limp and heavy . . . Good.

Scan your body for any muscle tension, starting with your head and going all the way down to your toes.

Release any tension in your face, head, and neck by letting your jaw become slack and your head feel heavy on your shoulders. Allow your shoulders to drop heavily. Take a deep breath and relax your chest and abdomen. Allow your arms and legs to feel heavy and to sink into the surface beneath you.

Now take a deep breath and become aware of any remaining tension in your body. As you breathe out, allow all the muscles of your body to sink heavily into the surface beneath you, becoming even more deeply relaxed . . . Good.

Imagine yourself walking along an old country road . . . the sun is warm on your back . . . the birds are singing . . . the air is calm and fragrant.

As you progress down the road, you come across an old gate . . . The gate creaks as you open it and go through.

You find yourself in an overgrown garden, flowers growing where they have seeded themselves, vines climbing over a fallen tree, green grass, shade trees.

Breathe deeply, smelling the flowers . . . listen to the birds and insects . . . feel the gentle breeze, warm against your skin.

As you walk leisurely up a gentle slope behind the garden, you come to a wooded area where the trees become denser, the sun is filtered through the leaves. The air feels mild and a bit cooler. You become aware of the sound and fragrance of a nearby brook. You breathe deeply of the cool and fragrant air several times, and with each breath, you feel more refreshed.

Soon, you come upon the brook. It is clear and clean as it tumbles over the rocks and some fallen logs. You follow the path along the brook for a way. The path takes you out into a sunlit clearing where you discover a small and picturesque waterfall . . . There is a rainbow in the mist . . .

You find a comfortable place to sit for a while, a perfect niche where you can feel completely relaxed.

You feel good as you allow yourself to just enjoy the warmth and solitude of this peaceful place.

It is now time to return. You walk back down the path, through the cool and fragrant trees, out into the sun-drenched overgrown garden . . . one last smell of the flowers, and out the creaky gate . . .

You leave this secret retreat for now and return down the country road. However, you know that you may visit this special place whenever you wish.

When you're ready, take three deep breaths, and open your eyes.

71

Visualization

This technique, also referred to as vivid imagery, is similar to guided imagery. It is another way of using your imagination to picture yourself any way you want, doing things you want to do. Visualization can be done in different ways and can be used for longer periods or while you are engaged in other activities.

One way to use visualization is to remember pleasant scenes from your past or create new scenes in your mind. It allows you to create more of your own images than does the guided imagery technique. For example, try to remember every detail of a special holiday or party that made you happy. Who was there? What happened? What did you talk about? You can do the same sort of thing by remembering a vacation.

In fact, visualization can also be used to plan the details of some future event. Try to fill in the details of a pleasant fantasy. For example, how would you spend a million dollars? What would be your ideal romantic encounter? What would your ideal home or garden look like? Where would you go and what would you do on your dream vacation?

Another form of visualization involves using your mind to think of symbols that represent the discomfort of pain felt in different parts of your body. For example, a painful joint might be red or a tight chest might have a constricting band around it. After forming these images, you then try to change them. The red color might fade until there is no more color, or the constricting band will stretch and stretch until it falls off.

Visualization is a useful technique to help you set and accomplish your personal goals (see Chapter 2). After you write your weekly action plan, take a few minutes to imagine yourself taking a walk, doing your exercises, or taking your medications. Here you are mentally rehearsing the steps you need to take in order to achieve your goal successfully.

Studies have shown that this technique can help people cope better with stressful situations, master skills, and accomplish personal goals. In fact, the people who have become skilled at visualization find they can actually reduce some of the discomfort and distress associated with symptoms by changing unpleasant images to pleasant ones.

All the relaxation techniques mentioned above can be used in conjunction with diaphragmatic breathing. This breathing technique is described in detail in Chapter 4, page 45; it can help you achieve a more relaxed state and keep your mind off any potential for shortness of breath.

72

Other Cognitive Strategies

While learning to relax is an important part of symptom management, other cognitive strategies can also be useful. These techniques, however, may require more practice than relaxation before you notice the benefits; they include distraction, positive thinking or self-talk, meditation, and prayer.

Distraction

Because our minds have trouble focusing on more than one thing at a time, we can lessen the intensity of symptoms by training our minds to focus attention on something other than our bodies and their sensations. This technique, called *distraction* or *attention refocusing*, is particularly helpful for those people who feel their symptoms are overwhelming, or worry that every bodily sensation might indicate a new or worsening symptom or health problem. (It is important to mention that with distraction you are not ignoring the symptoms, but choosing not to dwell on them.)

Distraction works best for short activities or episodes in which symptoms may be anticipated. For example, if you know climbing stairs will be painful or cause discomfort, or that falling asleep at night is difficult, you might try one of the following distraction techniques:

1. Make plans for exactly what you will do after the unpleasant activity passes. For example, if climbing stairs is uncomfortable or painful, think about what you need to do once you get to the top. If you have trouble falling asleep, try making plans for some future event, being as detailed as possible.

2. Think of a person's name, a bird, a flower, or whatever, for every letter of the alphabet. If you get stuck on one letter, go on to the next. (These are good distractions for pain as well as for sleep problems.)

3. Count backward from 1,000 or 100 by threes (e.g., 100, 97, 94, . . .).

4. To get through unpleasant daily chores (such as sweeping, mopping, or vacuuming), imagine your floor as a map of a country or continent. Try naming all the states, provinces, or countries, moving east to west or north to south. If geography does not appeal to you, imagine your favorite store and where each department is located.

5. Try to remember words to favorite songs or the events in an old story. There are, of course, a million variations to these examples, all of which help you to refocus attention away from your problem.

So far we have discussed short-term refocusing strategies that involve using only the mind for distraction. Distraction also works well for long-term projects or symptoms that tend to last longer, such as depression and some forms of chronic pain.

In these cases, the mind is not focused internally, but rather externally, on some type of activity. If you are somewhat depressed or have continuous unpleasant symptoms, find an activity that interests you and distract yourself from the problem. The activity can be almost anything, from gardening to cooking to reading or going to a movie, even doing volunteer work. One of the marks of a successful self-manager is that he or she has a variety of interests and always seems to be doing something.

74

Positive Thinking or Self-Talk—"I Know I Can"

All of us talk to ourselves all the time. For example, when waking up in the morning, we think, "I really don't want to get out of bed. I'm tired and don't want to go to work today." Or, at the end of an enjoyable evening, we think, "Gee, that was real fun. I should get out more often." These things we think or say to ourselves are referred to as "self-talk."

All of our self-talk is learned from others and becomes a part of us as we grow up. It comes in many forms, mostly negative. Negative self-statements are usually in the form of phrases that begin like these: "I just can't do . . ." "If only I could or didn't . . ." "I just don't have the energy . . . ." This type of self-talk represents the doubts and fears we have about ourselves in general, and about our abilities to deal with a disease and its symptoms in particular. Negative self-talk can worsen symptoms like pain, depression, and fatigue.

Because those things we learn in life influence our beliefs, attitudes, feelings, and actions, what we say to ourselves plays a major role in determining our success or failure in becoming good self-managers. Therefore, learning to make self-talk work *for* you instead of *against* you, by changing those negative statements to positive ones, will help you manage symptoms more effectively. This change, as with any habit, requires practice and includes the following steps:

1. Listen carefully to what you say *to* or *about* yourself, both out loud and silently. Then write down all the negative self-talk statements. Pay special attention to the things you say during times that are particularly difficult for you. For example, what do you say to yourself when getting up in the morning with pain, while doing those exercises you don't really like, or at those times when you are feeling blue?

2. Work on *changing* each negative statement you identified to a positive one, or find some positive statement to replace the negative one. Write these down. Positive statements should reflect the better you and your decision to be in control. For example, negative statements such as "I don't want to get up," "I'm too tired and I hurt," "I can't do the things I like anymore so why bother," or "I'm good for nothing," become positive messages such as "I have the energy to get up and do the things I enjoy," "I know I can do anything I believe I can," "People like me and I feel good about myself," or "Other people need and depend on me; I'm worthwhile."

3. *Read and rehearse* these positive statements, mentally or with another person. It is this conscious repetition or memorization of the positive self-talk that will help you replace those old, habitual negative statements.

4. *Practice these new statements in real situations.* This practice, along with time and patience, will help the new patterns of thinking become automatic.

Once established, positive thinking can be one of the most powerful tools you add to your self-management program; it will help you to manage symptoms as well as master the other skills discussed in this book.

As with exercise and other acquired skills, using your mind to manage your illness requires both practice and time before you will begin to notice the benefits. Thus, if you feel you are not accomplishing anything, don't give up. Be patient and keep on trying.

Mindfulness Meditation

There are many types of meditation. In fact, meditation is a part of most, if not every, religious or spiritual tradition. The purpose of meditation is to quiet the mind. It may also help the individual to quiet the body. For this reason, meditation is often a useful technique for managing stress and other symptoms such as pain, fatigue, or shortness of breath. Mindfulness meditation is one type of meditation that can be practiced by anyone. All that you need to begin is a quiet place and five or more minutes. Start by sitting in a chair with your feet flat on the floor and your hands in your lap or on your knees. If you wish and are able to, you can sit on the floor with crossed legs or in a more traditional yoga position. How you sit, however, does not matter.

The essence of mindfulness meditation is to concentrate fully on your breathing. It is best if you can do diaphragmatic or belly breathing, but you do not have to take deep breaths. It is important to keep your full attention on your breathing. Breathe in slowly; hold the breath for a moment, then breathe out slowly. At all times concentrate on your breathing.

While this seems fairly simple, you will soon find that your mind easily wanders. This is called "having a monkey mind." As soon as you notice that your mind is wandering, bring your attention back to your breathing. At first you may not be able to attend to your breathing for more than a minute or two. You will improve, however, with practice.

When you are doing this type of meditation, you may become very aware of your body. For example, your eye may itch or you may become uncomfortable in your sitting position. When this happens, first do nothing but pay attention to your breathing. In many cases you will find that the discomfort goes away. If it continues, however, scratch the itch or change your position. As you do this, pay full attention to what you are doing. With mindfulness meditation it is important to be fully aware of what you are doing at that moment!

Like all other self-management techniques, mindfulness meditation requires practice. You will not get results immediately; however, if you practice this for 15 to 30 minutes a day, four or five times a week, you will find that over time this can be a great symptom management tool.

Prayer

Over the years, many people with chronic illness have told us that prayer has been helpful in managing both the physical and emotional symptoms of their disease. In many ways, prayer is similar to some of the cognitive strategies discussed in this chapter. For some, it is a form of relaxation that helps reduce tension and anxiety. For others, it may be their method of distraction whereby they refocus their attention away from their symptoms. Regardless of the rationale, prayer is an important part of many people's self-management programs and remains the oldest of all symptom management techniques.

As we mentioned earlier, symptoms, their causes, and the ways they interact to affect your daily life can become a vicious cycle. Therefore, to successfully manage symptoms, it is important to identify them and their causes, in order to break this cycle.

Following are several key principles to remember from this and the previous chapter:

1. *Symptoms have many causes.* Thus, there are many ways to manage most symptoms. An understanding of the nature and varied causes of your symptoms and how these interact will help you to better manage them.

2. *Not all management techniques will work for everyone.* It is up to you to experiment and find out what works best for you. Be flexible. This includes trying different techniques and monitoring the results to determine which technique is most helpful for which symptom(s) and under what circumstances.

3. When trying to determine which techniques work best for you, remember that learning a new skill and gaining control of the situation take time. Therefore, *give yourself several weeks to practice* a new technique before you decide it is working for you.

4. As with exercise and other acquired skills, using your mind to manage your illness requires both practice and time before you notice the benefits. Thus, if you feel you are not accomplishing anything, *don't give up.* Be patient and keep on trying!

5. These techniques should not have negative effects. If you become frightened, angry, or depressed when using a cognitive technique, please do not continue to use it. Try another technique instead.

• • •

Suggested Further Reading

Borysenko, Joan. *Meditations for Relaxation and Stress Reduction.* Carlsbad, Calif.: Hayhouse, 1992.

Burns, David D. *The Feeling Good Handbook.* New York: NAL/Dutton, 1999.

Cousins, Norman. *Head First: The Biology of Hope and the Healing Power of the Human Spirit.* New York: E. P. Dutton, 1989.

Craze, Richard. *Teach Yourself Relaxation.* Chicago: Contemporary Publishing, 1998.

Davis, Martha, et al. *The Relaxation and Stress Reduction Workbook.* Oakland, Calif.: New Harbinger, 1988.

Dossey, Larry. *Prayer Is Good Medicine.* San Francisco: HarperCollins, 1996.

Kabat-Zinn, Jon. *Full Catastrophe Living: Using the Wisdom of Your Body to Face Stress, Pain and Illness*. New York: Dell Publishing Co., 1991.

Kabat-Zinn, Jon. *Wherever You Go, There You Are: Mindfulness Meditation in Everyday Life*. New York: Hyperion, 1995.

McKay, Matthew, and Patrick Fanning. *The Daily Relaxer*. Oakland, Calif.: New Harbinger, 1997.

McKay, Matthew, Patrick Fanning, Carole Honeychurch, and Catherine Sutker. *The Self-Esteem Companion: Simple Exercises to Help Challenge Your Inner Critic and Celebrate Your Personal Strengths*. Oakland, Calif.: New Harbinger, 1999.

Ornstein, Robert, and David Sobel. *Healthy Pleasures*. Reading, Mass.: Addison-Wesley, 1990.

Peale, Norman V. *The Powerful Way to Change Your Life*. New York: Ballantine Books, 1996.

Rolek, Michiko J. *Mental Fitness: Complete Workouts for Body, Mind and Soul*. New York: Weatherhill, 1996.

Sheller, Mary Dale. *Growing Older, Feeling Better in Body, Mind and Spirit*. Palo Alto, Calif.: Bull Publishing Co., 1993.

Siegel, Bernie S. *Love, Medicine and Miracles*. New York: Harper and Row, 1990.

78

CHAPTER
6

Exercising for Fun and Fitness

"The weakest and oldest among us can become some sort of athlete, but only the strongest can survive as spectators. Only the hardiest can withstand the perils of inertia, inactivity, and immobility."

J H Bland and S M Cooper,
Semin Arthritis Rheum:1984

REGULAR EXERCISE AND PHYSICAL ACTIVITY ARE VITAL to your physical and emotional health and can bring you fun and fitness at the same time. Having a chronic illness and growing older can make an active lifestyle seem far away. Some people have never been very active and others have given up leisure activities because of illness.

Unfortunately, long periods of inactivity in anyone can lead to weakness, stiffness, fatigue, poor appetite, high blood pressure, obesity, osteoporosis, constipation, and increased sensitivity to pain, anxiety, and depression. These problems occur from chronic illnesses, as well. So, it can be difficult to tell whether it is the illness, inactivity, or a combination of the two that is responsible for these problems. Although we do not have cures for many of these illnesses, yet, we do know the cure for inactivity—exercise!

Most people have a sense that exercising and being active is healthier and more satisfying than being inactive, but often have a hard time finding information and support to get started on a more active way of life.

Thanks to the knowledge gained from many people with chronic illnesses who have worked with health professionals in exercise research, we can now advise exercise for fun and fitness, as well as exercise for helping manage your illnesses and for making everyday activities less stressful.

In this chapter, you will learn how to improve your health and fitness and make wise exercise choices. However, this advice is not intended to take the place of therapeutic recommendations from your health care providers. If you've had an exercise plan prescribed for you that differs from the suggestions here, take this book to your doctor or therapist and ask what she or he thinks about this program. Later in this book, we will provide additional information and helpful exercise ideas for people with specific chronic illnesses.

Regular exercise benefits everyone, especially people with chronic health problems. Regular exercise improves levels of strength, energy, and self-confidence, and lessens anxiety and depression. Exercise can help maintain a good weight, which takes stress off weight-bearing joints and improves blood pressure, blood sugar, and blood fat levels. There is evidence that regular exercise can help to "thin" the blood, or prevent blood clots, which is one of the reasons exercise can be of particular benefit to people with heart disease, cerebrovascular disease, and peripheral vascular disease.

In addition, strong muscles can help people with arthritis to protect their joints by improving stability and absorbing shock. Regular exercise also helps nourish joints and keep cartilage and bone healthy. Regular exercise has been shown to help people with chronic lung disease improve endurance and reduce shortness of breath (and trips to the emergency room!). Many people with claudication (leg pain from severe atherosclerotic blockages in the arteries of the lower extremities) can walk farther without leg pain after undertaking a regular exercise program. Studies of people with heart disease who exercise in cardiac rehabilitation programs suggest that exercise may even increase life expectancy. Regular exercise is an important part of controlling blood sugar levels, losing weight, and reducing the risks of cardiovascular complications for people with diabetes.

The good news is that it doesn't take hours of painful, sweat-soaked exercise to achieve most of these health benefits. Even short periods of gentle physical activity can significantly improve health and fitness, reduce disease risks, and boost your mood.

Exercise reconditions your body, helping to restore function previously lost to disuse and illness. This will help you improve your health, feel better, and manage your chronic illness better. Feeling more in control and less at the mercy of your chronic illness is one of the biggest and best benefits of becoming an exercise self-manager.

Developing an Active Lifestyle

OK, so you want to be more physically active. One way is to set aside a special time for a formal exercise program, involving such planned activities as walking, jogging, swimming, tennis, aerobic dance, exercise to an exercise videotape, and so on. But don't underestimate the value and importance of just being more physically active throughout the day as you carry out your usual activities. Both can be helpful.

The formal programs are usually more visible and get more attention. But being more physical in everyday life can also pay off. Consider taking the stairs a floor or two instead of waiting impatiently for a slow elevator. Park and walk several blocks to work or to the store instead of circling the parking lot looking for the perfect, up-close parking space. Mow the lawn, work in the garden, or just get up once in a while and walk around the house.

These types of daily activities, often not viewed as "exercise," can add up to significant health benefits. Recent studies show that even small amounts of daily activity can raise fitness levels, decrease heart disease risk, and boost mood . . . and the activities can be pleasurable, enjoyable ones! Playing with the children, dancing, gardening, bowling, golf . . . all these enjoyable activities can make a big difference. One person commented that she *never* exercised. When asked why she went square-dancing several times a week she replied, "Oh, that's not exercise, that's fun." The average day is filled with excellent opportunities to be more physical.

Developing an Exercise Program

For many people, however, a more formal exercise program can be helpful. This usually involves setting aside a period of time, at least several times a week, to deliberately focus on increasing fitness. A complete, balanced exercise program should help you improve these three aspects of fitness:

1. *Flexibility.* This refers to the ability of the joints and muscles to move comfortably through a full, normal range of motion. Limited flexibility can cause pain, increase risk of injury, and make muscles less efficient. Flexibility tends to diminish with inactivity, age, and certain diseases, but you can increase or maximize your flexibility by doing gentle stretching exercises like those described later in Chapter 7.

2. *Strength.* Muscles need to be exercised to maintain their strength. With inactivity, muscles tend to weaken and shrink (atrophy). The weaker the muscles get, the less we feel like using them, and the more inactive we tend to become, creating a vicious circle. Much of the disability and lack of mobility for

81

people with chronic illness is due to muscle weakness. This weakness can be reversed with a program of gradually increasing exercise.

3. *Endurance.* Our ability to sustain activity depends on certain vital capacities. The heart and lungs must work efficiently to distribute oxygen-rich blood to the muscles. The muscles must be conditioned to use the oxygen.

Aerobic (meaning "with oxygen") exercise improves this cardiovascular and muscular conditioning. This type of exercise uses the large muscles of your body in a rhythmical, continuous activity. The most effective activities involve your whole body: walking, swimming, dancing, mowing the lawn, and so on. Aerobic exercise improves cardiovascular fitness, lessens heart attack risk, and helps control weight. Aerobic exercise also promotes a sense of well-being . . . easing depression and anxiety, promoting restful sleep, and improving mood and energy levels.

Your Fitness Program

A complete fitness program combines exercises to improve each of the three aspects of fitness: flexibility, strength, and endurance. Chapter 7 explains and illustrates a number of flexibility and strengthening exercises. Chapter 8 contains information about endurance or aerobic exercise. If you haven't exercised regularly in some time, or have pain, stiffness, shortness of breath, or weakness that interferes with your daily activities, it is a good idea to discuss your ideas about increasing your exercise with your health care providers. Begin your fitness program by choosing a number of flexibility and strengthening exercises that you are willing to do every day or every other day. Once you are able to comfortably exercise for at least 10 minutes at a time, you are ready to start adding some endurance or aerobic activities.

Many people wonder how to choose the right exercises and how to know what's best for them. The truth is that the best exercises for you are the ones that will help you do what you want to do. Often, the most important decision to start a successful fitness program is to choose a goal (something you want to do) that exercise can help you reach. Once you have a goal in mind, it is much easier to choose exercises that make sense to you. There is no doubt that we all are more successful exercisers if we know where we want exercise to take us. If you don't see how exercise can be helpful to you, it is hard to get excited about adding just another task to our days.

Choose Your Goal and Make a Plan

1. **Choose a goal** that you want to do but don't or can't do now because of some physical reason. For example, you might want to enjoy a shopping or fishing trip with your friends, mow the lawn, or take a family vacation.

2. **Think about why you can't or don't do it or enjoy doing it now.** It might be that you get tired before everybody else, that it's too hard to get up from a low chair or bench, that climbing steps is painful or makes your legs tired, or that your shoulders are too weak or stiff to cast your fishing line or stow a carry-on bag.

3. **Decide what about your abilities makes it difficult to do what you want.** For example, if getting up from a low seat is difficult, you may realize that your hips, knees, or joints are stiff and that your leg muscles are weak. In this case, look for flexibility and strengthening exercises for hips and knees. If you decide a major problem is that your shoulders are stiff and your arms too weak to handle a carry-on bag for a plane trip, choose flexibility and strengthening exercises for your shoulders and arms.

4. **Design your exercise plan.** Choose no more than 10–12 exercises at first. Start by doing 3–5 repetitions of each and review the information in Chapter 7. As you get comfortable, you can increase repetitions and kinds of exercise. If you want to improve your endurance, read over Chapter 8 about aerobic exercise. Start off with short periods and build up gradually. Health and fitness take time to build, but every day you exercise you are healthier and on your way to fitness. That's why it's so important to make sure you keep it up.

What Are Your Exercise Barriers?

Health and fitness make sense. Yet, when faced with actually being more physically active, most people can come up with scores of excuses, concerns, and worries. These barriers can prevent us from even taking the first step. Here are some common barriers and possible solutions:

"I don't have enough time." Everyone has the same amount of time. We just choose to use it differently. It's a matter of priorities. Some find a lot of time for television, but nothing to spare for fitness. It doesn't really take a lot of time.

Even five minutes a day is a good start, and it's much better than no physical activity. You may be able to combine activities, like watching television while pedaling a stationary bicycle, or arranging "walking meetings" to discuss business or family matters.

"I'm too tired." When you're out of shape, you feel listless and tend to tire easily. Then you don't exercise because you're tired, and this becomes yet another vicious cycle. You have to break out of the "too tired" cycle. Regular physical activity increases your stamina and gives you more energy to do the things you like. As you get back into shape, you will recognize the difference between feeling listless or "out of shape" and feeling physically tired.

"I'm too old." You're never too old for some type of physical activity. No matter what your level of fitness is or your age, you can always find some ways to increase activity, energy, and sense of well-being. To date our oldest self-manager has been 99. Fitness is especially important as we age.

"I'm too sick." It may be true that you are too sick for a vigorous or strenuous exercise program, but you can usually find some ways to be more active. Remember, you can exercise one minute at a time, several times a day. The enhanced physical fitness can help you better cope with your illness and prevent further problems.

"I get enough exercise." This may be true, but for most people, their jobs and daily activities do not provide enough sustained exercise to keep them fully fit and energetic.

"Exercise is boring." You can make it more interesting and fun. Exercise with other people. Entertain yourself with a headset and musical tapes or listen to the radio. Vary your activities and your walking routes.

"Exercise is painful." The old saying "No pain, no gain" is simply wrong and out-of-date. Recent evidence shows significant health benefits come from gentle, low-intensity enjoyable physical activity. You may sweat, or feel a bit short of breath, but if you feel more pain when you finish than before you started, take a close look at what you are doing. More than likely you are either exercising improperly or overdoing it for your particular condition. Talk with your instructor, therapist, or doctor. You may simply need to be less vigorous or change the type of exercise that you're doing.

"I'm too embarrassed." For some, the thought of donning a skintight, designer exercise outfit and trotting around in public is delightful, but for others it is downright distressing. Fortunately, as we'll describe, the options for physical activity range from exercise in the privacy of your own home to group social activities. You should be able to find something that suits you.

"I'm afraid I'll have a heart attack." In most cases, the risk of a heart attack may be greater for those who are not physically active than for those who exercise

84

regularly. But if you are worried about this, check with your doctor. Especially if your illness is under control, it's probably safer to exercise than *not* to exercise

"It's too cold, it's too hot, it's too dark, etc." If you are flexible, and vary your type of exercise, you can generally work around the changes in weather that make certain types of exercise more difficult. Consider indoor activities like stationary bicycling or mall walking.

"I'm afraid I won't be able to do it right or be successful. I'm afraid I'll fail." Many people don't start a new project because they are afraid they will fail or not be able to finish it successfully. If you feel this way about starting an exercise program, remember two things. First, whatever activities you are able to do—no matter how short or "easy"—will be much better for you than doing nothing. Be proud of what you *have* done, not guilty about what you *haven't* done. Second, new projects often seem overwhelming—until we get started and learn to enjoy each day's adventures and successes.

Perhaps you have come up with some other barriers. The human mind is incredibly creative. But you can turn that creativity to your advantage by using it to come up with even better ways to refute the excuses and develop positive attitudes about exercise and fitness. If you get stuck, ask others for suggestions, or try some of the self-talk suggestions in Chapter 5.

Preparing to Exercise

Figuring out how to make the commitment of time and energy to regular exercise is a challenge for everyone. If you have a chronic illness, you have even more challenges. You must take precautions and find a safe and comfortable program. Even with a chronic illness, most people can do some kind of aerobic exercise.

If your illness is not fairly stable, if you have been inactive for more than six months, or if you have questions about starting an aerobic exercise program, it is best to check with your doctor or therapist first. Take this book with you when you discuss your exercise ideas, or prepare a list of your specific questions.

People with arthritis, for example, should understand how to adapt their exercise to changes in their arthritis and joint problems. People with heart disease or lung disease should generally not "exercise through" potentially serious symptoms, such as chest pain, palpitations (irregular heartbeats), shortness of breath, or excessive fatigue. They should notify their physicians of any significant worsening of their usual symptoms or if new symptoms appear. Resumption of exercise should begin only after getting the physician's clearance to do so. Also, don't exercise when you are experiencing flu symptoms, an upset stomach, diarrhea, or other acute illnesses. Learning how much to push yourself while exercising, without doing "too much," is especially important.

We hope that this chapter will help you gain knowledge to meet these challenges and enjoy the benefits of physical fitness. Start by learning your individual needs and limits. If possible, talk with your doctor and other health professionals who understand your kind of chronic illness. Get their ideas about special exercise needs and precautions. Read Chapter 9 in this book. Learn to be aware of your body, and plan activities accordingly.

86

Respect your body. If you feel acutely ill, don't exercise. If you can't comfortably complete your warm-up period of flexibility and strengthening exercises, then don't try to do more vigorous conditioning exercises. Your personal exercise program should be based on *your* current level of health and fitness, *your* goals and desires, *your* abilities and special needs, and *your* likes and dislikes. Deciding to improve your fitness, and feeling the satisfaction of success, has nothing to do with competition or comparing yourself to others.

Opportunities in Your Community

Most people who exercise regularly do so with at least one other person. Two or more people can keep each other motivated, and a whole class can build a feeling of camaraderie. On the other hand, exercising alone gives you the most freedom. You may feel that there are no classes that would work for you or no buddy with whom to exercise. If so, start your own program; as you progress, you may find that these feelings change.

The Arthritis Foundation sponsors exercise programs taught by trained instructors and developed specifically for people with arthritis. The heart and lung associations and diabetes organizations are excellent resources for people who have had heart disease, a stroke, lung disease, or diabetes. Consult your local chapter or branch of the appropriate agency.

Most communities now offer a variety of exercise classes, including special programs for people over 50, adaptive exercises, mall walking, fitness trails, tai chi, yoga, and others. Check with the local Y, community and senior centers, parks and recreation programs, adult education, and community colleges. There is a great deal of variation in the content of these programs, as well as in the professional experience of the exercise staff. By and large, the classes are inexpensive, and those in charge of planning are responsive to people's needs.

Hospitals commonly offer medically supervised exercise classes for people with heart or lung disease (cardiac or pulmonary rehabilitation classes). Occasionally, people with other chronic illnesses can be included as well. These programs tend to be more expensive than other community classes, but there is the advantage of medical supervision, if that's important to you.

Health and fitness clubs usually offer aerobic studios, weight training, cardiovascular equipment, and sometimes a heated pool. For all these services they charge membership fees, which can be high. Ask about low-impact, beginners, and over-50 exercise classes, both in the aerobic studio and in the pool. Gyms that emphasize weight lifting generally don't have the programs or personnel to help you with a flexible, overall fitness program. These are some qualities you should look for:

87

1. Classes designed for *moderate and low-intensity* exercise and for beginners. You should be able to observe classes and participate in at least one class before signing up and paying.
2. Instructors with *qualifications and experience.* Knowledgeable instructors are more likely to understand special needs and be willing and able to work with you.
3. Membership policies that allow you to pay only for a session of classes or let you "freeze" membership at times when you can't participate. Some fitness facilities offer *different rates* depending on how many services you use.
4. Facilities that are *easy to get to, park near, and enter.* Dressing rooms and exercise sites should be accessible and safe, with professional staff on site.
5. A pool that allows *"free swim" times* when the water isn't crowded. Also, find out the policy about children in the pool; small children playing and making noise may not be compatible with your program.
6. Staff and other members whom you *feel comfortable* being around.

One last note: There are many excellent videotapes for use at home. These vary in intensity, from very gentle chair exercises to more strenuous aerobic exercise. Ask your doctor, therapist, or voluntary agency for suggestions, or review the tapes yourself.

Putting Your Program Together

The best way to enjoy and stick with your exercise program is to *suit yourself!* Choose what you want to do, a place where you feel comfortable, and an exercise time that fits your schedule. A woman who wants to have dinner on the table at 6 won't stick with an exercise program that requires her to leave home for a 5 o'clock class. A retired man who enjoys lunch with friends and an afternoon nap is wise to choose an early- or mid-morning exercise time.

Pick two or three activities you think you would enjoy and that wouldn't put undue stress on your body. Choose activities that can be easily worked into your daily routine. If an activity is new to you, try it out before going to the expense of buying equipment or joining a health club. By having more than one exercise, you can keep active while adapting to vacations, seasons, and changing problems with your condition. Variety also helps keep you from getting bored.

Having fun and enjoying yourself are benefits of exercise that often go unmentioned. Too often we think of exercise as serious business. However, most people who stick with a program do so because they enjoy it. *They think of their exercise as recreation rather than a chore.* Start off with success in mind. Allow yourself time to get used to new experiences and meet new people. You'll probably find that you look forward to exercise.

Some well-meaning health professionals can make it hard for a person with a chronic illness to stick to an exercise program. You may have been told simply to "exercise more on your own." The "how" and "when" of that exercise plan, in fact, may have been left entirely up to you. No wonder so many people never start or give up so quickly! Not many of us would make a commitment to do something we don't fully understand. Experience, practice, and success help us establish a habit. Follow the self-management steps in Chapter 2 to make beginning your program easier.

1. *Keep your exercise goal in mind.* Review "Choose Your Goal and Make a Plan" earlier in this chapter.

2. *Choose exercises you want to do.* Combine activities that move you toward your goal and those recommended by your health professionals. Select exercises and activities from the next two chapters to get started.

3. *Choose the time and place to exercise.* Tell your family and friends your plan.

4. *Make an action plan with yourself.* Decide how long you'll stick with these particular exercises. Six to eight weeks is a reasonable time commitment for a new program.

5. *Make an exercise diary or calendar,* whichever suits you. A diary or journal will let you record more information. Some people enjoy having a record of what they did and how they felt. For others, a simple calendar on which to note an exercise session is plenty of paperwork. Choose what you like; the point is to have fun and enjoy being active.

6. *Do some self-tests to keep track of your progress.* You will find these at the end of the next two chapters. Record the date and results of the ones you choose.

7. *Start your program.* Remember to begin gradually and proceed slowly, especially if you haven't exercised in a while.

8. *Repeat the self-tests* at regular intervals, record the results, and check the changes.

9. *Revise your program.* At the end of your 6–8 weeks, decide what you liked, what worked, and what made exercising difficult. Modify your program and contract for another few weeks. You may decide to change some exercises, the place or time you exercise, or your exercise partner(s).

10. *Reward yourself for a job well done.* Many people who start an exercise program find that the rewards come with improved fitness and endurance. Being able to enjoy family outings, a refreshing walk, or trips to the store, the library, a concert, or a museum are great rewards to look forward to.

Keeping It Up

If you haven't exercised recently, you'll undoubtedly experience some new feelings and discomfort in the early days. It's normal to feel muscle tension and possible tenderness around joints, and to be a little more tired in the evenings. *Muscle or joint pain that lasts more than two hours after the exercise, or feeling tired into the next day, means that you probably did too much too fast. Don't stop;* just exercise less vigorously or for a shorter amount of time the next day.

When you do aerobic exercise, it's natural to feel your heart beat faster, your breathing speed up, and your body get warmer. However, feeling chest pain, excessive shortness of breath, nausea, or dizziness is not what you want. If this happens to you, stop exercising and discontinue your program until you check with your doctor. (See Table 6.1.)

People who have a chronic illness often have *additional sensations* to sort out. It can be difficult at first to figure out whether it is the illness or the exercise or both that is causing them. Talking to someone else with the illness who has had experience starting a new exercise program can be a big help. Once you've sorted out the new sensations, you'll be able to exercise with confidence.

Expect setbacks. During the first year, people average two to three interruptions in their exercise schedule, often because of minor injuries or illnesses unrelated to

Table 6.1 *Advice for Exercise Problems*

Problem	Advice
Irregular or very rapid heartbeats	Stop exercising. Check your pulse. Are the beats regular or irregular? How fast is your heartbeat? Make a note of these and discuss this information with your doctor before exercising again.
Pain, tightness, or pressure in the chest, jaw, arms, neck, or back	Stop exercising. Talk with your doctor. Don't exercise until it has been cleared by your doctor.
Unusual, extreme shortness of breath, persisting 10 minutes after you exercise	Notify your doctor and get clearance before exercising again.
Light-headedness, dizziness, fainting, cold sweat, or confusion	Lie down with your feet up, or sit down and put your head between your legs. If it happens more than once, check with your doctor before you exercise again.
Excessive tiredness after exercise, especially if you're still tired 24 hours after you exercise	Don't exercise so vigorously next time. If the excessive tiredness persists, check with your doctor. Talk to your doctor before you exercise again.

their exercise. You may find yourself sidelined or derailed temporarily. Don't be discouraged. Try a different activity or simply rest. When you are feeling better, resume your program, but begin at a lower, more gentle level. As a rule of thumb, it will take you the same amount of time to get back into shape as you were out. For instance, if you missed three weeks, it may take at least that long to get back to your previous level. Go slowly. Be kind to yourself. You're in this for the long haul.

Think of your head as the coach and your body as your team. For success, all parts of the team need attention. Be a good coach. *Encourage and praise yourself.* Design "plays" you feel your team can execute successfully. Choose places that are safe and hospitable. A good coach knows his or her team, sets good goals, and helps the team succeed. A good coach is loyal. A good coach does not belittle, nag, or make anyone feel guilty. Be a good coach to your team.

Besides a good coach, everyone needs an enthusiastic cheerleader or two. Of course, you can be your own cheerleader, but being both coach and cheerleader is a lot to do. Successful exercisers usually have at least one *family member* or close friend who actively *supports* their exercise habit. Your cheerleader can exercise with you, help you get other chores done, praise your accomplishments, or just consider your exercise time when making plans. Sometimes cheerleaders pop up by themselves, but don't be bashful about asking for a hand.

With exercise experience you develop a sense of control over yourself and your chronic illness. You learn how to *alternate your activities to fit your day-to-day needs.* You know when to do less and when to do more. You know that a change in symptoms or a period of inactivity is usually only temporary and doesn't have to be devastating. You know you have the tools to get back on track again.

Give your exercise plan a chance to succeed. Set reasonable goals and enjoy your success. Stay motivated. When it comes to your personal fitness program, sticking with it and doing it your way makes you a definite winner.

Community Resource Detective's Kit

Exercising for Future Fitness

Heart Association
Lung Association
Diabetes Association
Arthritis Foundation/Society
Diabetes organizations
Other disease-specific organizations
Community colleges, YMCA–YWCA
Hospitals, health care organizations
Parks and recreation departments
Adult education

• • •

Suggested Further Reading

Green, Tamara. *Exercise Is Fun! (Good Health Guides)*. Gareth Stevens, 1998.

Rizzo, Terrie. *Fresh Start: The Stanford Medical School Health and Fitness Program*. San Francisco: KQED Books, 1996. Order from: Stanford University HIP, 1000 Welch Road, Palo Alto, CA 94394. Call 650-723-9649 for information.

White, Martha. *Water Exercise: 78 Safe and Effective Exercises for Fitness and Therapy*. Champaign, Ill.: Human Kinetics, 1995.

92

CHAPTER
7

Exercising for Flexibility and Strength:
Warm-Up/Cool-Down

YOU CAN USE THE EXERCISES IN THIS CHAPTER IN SEVERAL WAYS: to get in shape for more vigorous aerobic exercise, on days when you don't do aerobic exercise, and as part of your warm-up and cool-down routines. Choose exercises to build a strengthening and flexibility program for the whole body.

The exercises are arranged in order from the head and neck down to the toes. Most of the upper-body exercises may be done either sitting or standing. Exercises done lying down can be performed on the floor or on a firm mattress. We have labeled the exercises that are particularly important for good posture "VIP" *(Very Important for Posture)*.

You might enjoy creating a routine of exercises that flow together. Arrange them so that you don't have to get up and down too often. Exercising to gentle, rhythmical music can also add to your enjoyment.

These helpful tips apply to all the exercises that follow:

- *Move slowly and gently.* Do not bounce or jerk.
- To loosen tight muscles and limber up stiff joints, stretch *just until you feel tension,* hold for 5 to 10 seconds, and then relax.
- *Don't push your body until it hurts.* Stretching should feel good, not painful.
- *Start with no more than 5 repetitions* of any exercise. Take at least *2 weeks* to increase to 10 repetitions.
- Always do the *same number* of exercises for your left side as for your right.

- *Breathe naturally.* Do not hold your breath. Count out loud to make sure you are breathing easily.
- If you feel increased symptoms that last more than *2 hours* after exercising, next time do fewer repetitions, or eliminate an exercise that seems to be causing the symptoms. *Don't quit exercising.*
- *All exercises can be adapted for individual needs.* The following exercises are designed and pictured to include both sides of the body and full range of motion. If you are limited by muscle weakness or joint tightness, go ahead and do the exercise as completely as you can. ***The benefit of doing an exercise comes from moving toward a certain position, not from being able to complete the movement perfectly.*** In some cases you may find that after a while you can complete the movement. Other times, you will continue to perform your own version.

Neck Exercises

1. Heads Up *(VIP)*

This exercise relieves jaw, neck, and upper back tension or pain, and is the start of good posture. You can do it while driving, sitting at a desk, sewing, reading, or exercising. Just sit or stand straight and gently slide your chin back. Keep looking forward as your chin moves backward. You'll feel the back of your neck lengthen and straighten. To help, put your finger on your nose and then draw straight back from your finger. (Don't worry about a little double chin—you really look much better with your neck straight!)

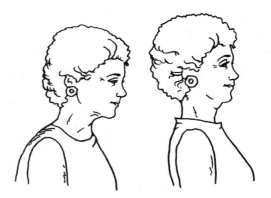

Clues for finding the correct position:

1. Ear over shoulder, *not* out in front.
2. Head balanced over neck and trunk, *not* in the lead.
3. Back of neck more vertical, not leaning forward.
4. Bit of double chin.

2. Neck Stretch

In heads-up position (Exercise 1) and with your shoulders relaxed:

a. Turn slowly to look over your right shoulder. Then turn slowly to look over your left shoulder.

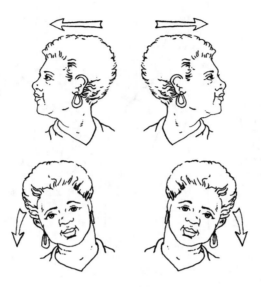

b. Tilt your head to the right and then to the left. Move your ear toward your shoulder. Do *not* move your shoulder up to your ear.

Don't do these exercises if they cause neck pain, or pain or numbness in your arms or hands.

Hand and Wrist Exercises

A good place to do hand exercises is at a table that supports your forearms. Do them after washing dishes, after bathing, or when taking a break from handwork. Your hands are warmer and more limber at these times.

3. Thumb Walk

Holding your wrist straight, form the letter "O" by lightly touching your thumb to each fingertip. After each "O," straighten and spread your fingers. Use the other hand to help if needed.

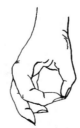
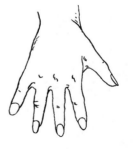

Shoulder Exercises

4. Good Morning Stretch

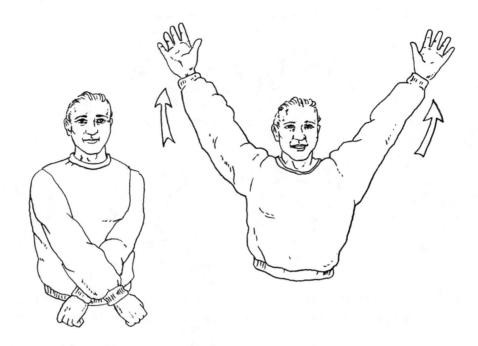

Start with hands in gentle fists, palms turned away from you, and wrists crossed. Breathe in and extend fingers while you uncross your arms and reach up as high as you can. Breathe out and relax.

5. Wand Exercise

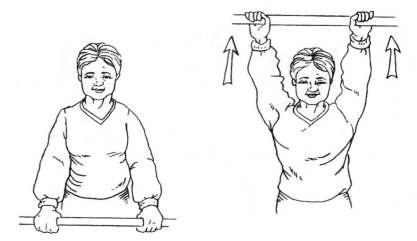

If one or both of your shoulders are tight or weak, you may want to give yourself a "helping hand." This shoulder exercise and the next allow the arms to help each other.

Use a cane, yardstick, or mop handle as your wand. Place one hand on each end and raise the wand as high overhead as possible. You might try this in front of the mirror. This wand exercise can be done standing, sitting, or lying down.

6. Pat and Reach

This double-duty exercise helps increase flexibility and strength for both shoulders. Raise one arm up over your head, and bend your elbow to pat yourself on the back. Move your other arm to your back, bend your elbow, and reach up toward the other hand. Can your fingertips touch? Relax and switch arm positions. Can you touch on that side? For most people, one position will work better than the other.

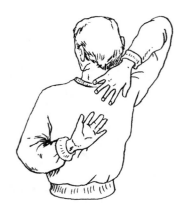

7. Shoulder Blade Pinch (VIP)

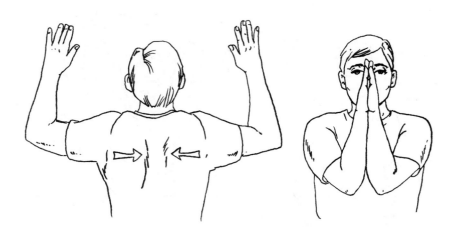

This is a good exercise to strengthen the middle and upper back and to stretch the chest. Sit or stand with your head in heads-up position (Exercise 1) and your shoulders relaxed. Raise your arms out to the sides with elbows bent. Pinch your shoulder blades together by moving your elbows as far back as you can. Hold briefly, then slowly move your arms forward to touch elbows. If this position is uncomfortable, lower your arms or rest your hands on your shoulders.

Back and Abdominal Exercises

8. Knee to Chest Stretch

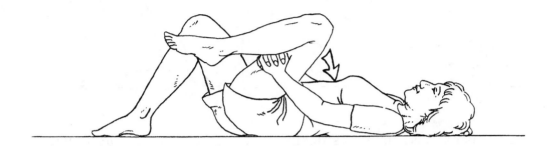

For a low back stretch, lie on the floor with knees bent and feet flat. Bring one knee toward your chest, using your hands to help. Hold your knee near your chest for 10 seconds and lower the leg slowly. Repeat with the other knee. You can also tuck both legs at the same time if you wish. Relax and enjoy the stretch.

9. Pelvic Tilt *(VIP)*

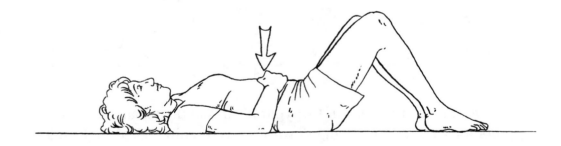

This is an excellent exercise for the low back. Lie on your back with knees bent, feet flat. Place your hands on your abdomen. Flatten the small of your back against the floor by tightening your stomach muscles and your buttocks. It helps to imagine bringing your pubic bone to your chin, or trying to pull your tummy in enough to zip a tight pair of trousers. Hold the tilt for 5 to 10 seconds. Relax. Arch your back slightly. Relax and repeat the Pelvic Tilt. Keep breathing. Count the seconds out loud. Once you've mastered the Pelvic Tilt lying down, practice it sitting, standing, and walking.

10. Back Lift (VIP)

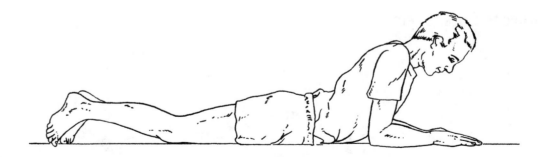

100

a. This exercise improves flexibility along your spine. Lie on your stomach and rise up onto your forearms. Keep your back relaxed, and keep your stomach and hips down. If this is comfortable, straighten your elbows. Breathe naturally and relax for at least 10 seconds. If you have moderate to severe low back pain, do not do this exercise unless it has been specifically prescribed for you.

b. To strengthen back muscles, lie on your stomach with your arms

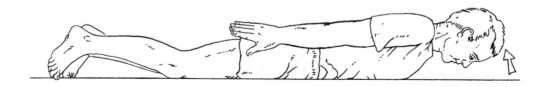

at your side or overhead. Lift your head, shoulders, and arms. Do *not* look up. Keep looking down with your chin tucked in. Count out loud as you hold for a count of 10. Relax. You can also lift your legs, instead of your head and shoulders, off the floor

Lifting both ends of your body at once is a fairly strenuous exercise. It may not be helpful for a person with back pain.

11. Low Back Rock and Roll

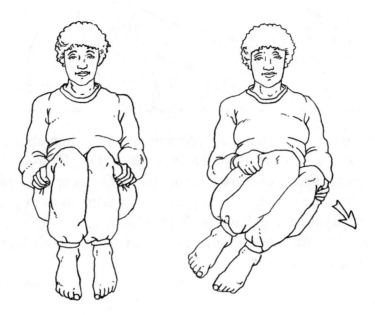

Lie on your back and pull your knees up to your chest with your hands behind the thighs. Rest in this position for 10 seconds, then gently roll knees from one side to the other, rocking your hips back and forth. Keep your upper back and shoulders flat on the ground.

12. Curl-Up

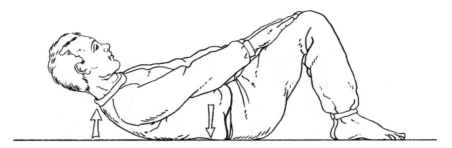

A curl-up, as shown here, is a good way to strengthen abdominal muscles. Lie on your back, *knees bent,* feet flat. Do the Pelvic Tilt (Exercise 9). Slowly curl up to raise your head and shoulders. Uncurl back down, or hold for 10 seconds and slowly lower. Breathe out as you curl up, and breathe in as you go back down. Do *not* hold your breath. If you have neck problems, or if your neck hurts when you do this exercise, try the next one instead. *Never* tuck your feet under a chair or have someone hold your feet!

13. Roll-Out

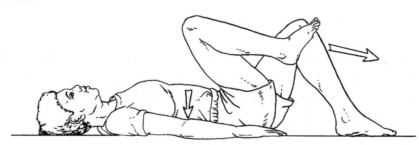

This is another good abdominal strengthener, and easy on the neck. Use it instead of the curl-up, or, if neck pain is not a problem, do them both.

- Lie on your back with knees bent and feet flat. Do the Pelvic Tilt (Exercise 9), and hold your lower back firmly against the floor.
- Slowly and carefully, move one leg away from your chest as you straighten your knee. Move your leg out until you feel your lower back start to arch. When this happens, tuck your knee back to your chest. Reset your pelvic tilt and roll your leg out again. Breathe out as your leg rolls out. Do *not* hold your breath. Repeat with the other leg.

You are strengthening your abdominal muscles by holding your pelvic tilt against the weight of your leg. As you get stronger, you'll be able to straighten your legs out farther and move both legs together.

Hip and Leg Exercises

14. Straight Leg Raises

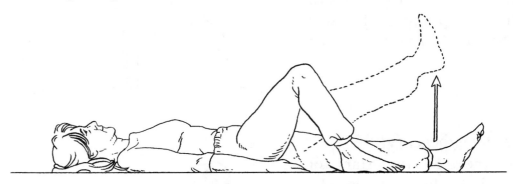

This exercise strengthens the muscles that bend the hip and straighten the knee. Lie on your back, knees bent, feet flat. Straighten one leg. Tighten the muscle on the top of that thigh, and straighten the knee as much as possible. Keeping the knee straight, raise your leg one to two feet (about 50 cm) off the ground. Do not arch your back. Hold your leg up and count out loud for 10 seconds. Relax. Repeat with the other leg.

15. Hip Hooray

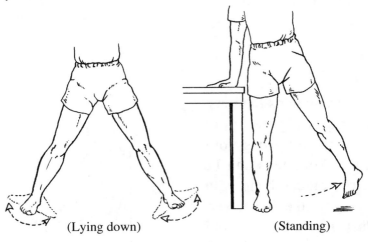

(Lying down)   (Standing)

This exercise can be done standing or lying on your back. If you lie down, spread your legs as far apart as possible. Roll your legs and feet out like a duck, then in to be pigeon-toed, move your legs back together. If you are standing, move one leg out to your side as far as you can. Lead out with the heel and in with the toes. Hold onto a counter for support.

16. Back Kick *(VIP)*

This exercise increases the backward mobility and strength of your hip. Hold onto a counter for support. Move the leg up and back, knee straight. Stand tall, and do not lean forward.

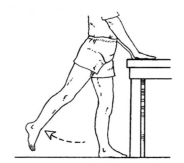

17. Knee Strengthener *(VIP)*

Strong knees are important for walking and standing comfortably. This exercise strengthens the knee. Sitting in a chair, straighten the knee by tightening up the muscle on top of your thigh. Place your hand on your thigh and feel the muscle work. If you wish, make circles with your toes. As your knee strengthens, see if you can build up to holding your leg out for 30 seconds. Count out loud. Do *not* hold your breath.

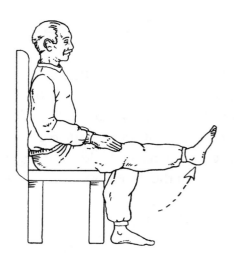

18. Power Knees

This exercise strengthens the muscles that bend and straighten your knee. Sit in a chair and cross your legs at the ankles. Your legs can be almost straight, or you can bend your knees as much as you like. Try several positions. Push forward with your back leg, and press backward with your front leg. Exert pressure evenly so that your legs do not move. Hold and count out loud for 10 seconds. Relax. Change leg positions. Be sure to keep breathing. Repeat.

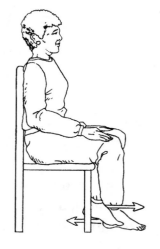

19. Ready-Go *(VIP)*

Stand with one leg slightly in front of the other in the position of having your heel on the floor ready to take a step with the front foot. Now tighten the muscles on the front of your thigh, making your knee firm and straight. Hold to count of 10. Relax. Repeat with the other leg.

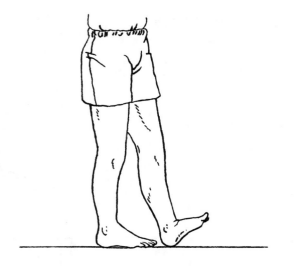

105

20. Hamstring Stretch

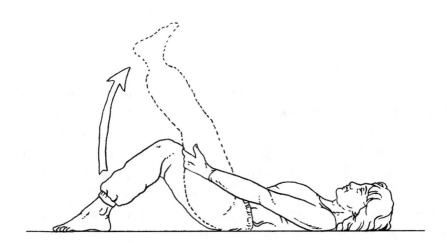

Do the self-test for hamstring tightness (page 110) to see if you need to do this exercise. If you have unstable knees, or "back knee" (a knee that curves backward when you stand up), do not do this exercise.

If you do have tight hamstrings, lie on your back, knees bent, feet flat. Grasp one leg at a time behind the thigh. Holding the leg out at arm's length, slowly straighten the knee. Hold the leg as straight as you can as you count to 10. You should feel a slight stretch at the back of your knee and thigh.

Be careful with this exercise. It's easy to overstretch and be sore.

21. Achilles Stretch

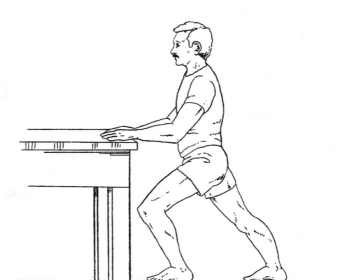

106

This exercise helps maintain flexibility in the Achilles tendon, the large tendon you feel at the back of your ankle. Good flexibility helps reduce the risk of injury, calf discomfort, and heel pain. The Achilles Stretch is especially helpful for cooling down after walking or cycling, and for people who get cramps in the calf muscles. If you have trouble with standing balance or spasticity (muscle jerks), you can do a seated version of this exercise. Sit in a chair with feet flat on the floor. Keep your heel on the floor and slowly slide your foot (one foot at a time) back to bend your ankle and feel some tension on the back of your calf.

Stand at a counter or against a wall. Place one foot in front of the other, toes pointing forward and heels on the ground. Lean forward, bend the knee of the forward leg, and keep the back knee straight, heel down. You will feel a good stretch in the calf. Hold the stretch for 10 seconds. Do *not* bounce. Move gently.

It's easy to get sore doing this exercise. If you've worn shoes with high heels for a long time, be particularly careful.

22. Tiptoes

This exercise will help strengthen your calf muscles and make walking, climbing stairs, and standing less tiring. It may also improve your balance. Hold on to a counter or table for support and raise up on your tiptoes. Hold for 10 seconds. Lower slowly. How high you go is not as important as keeping your balance and controlling your ankles. It is easier to do both legs at the same time. If your feet are too sore to do this standing, start doing it while sitting down. If this exercise makes your ankle jerk, leave it out, and talk to your therapist about other ways to strengthen these calf muscles if needed.

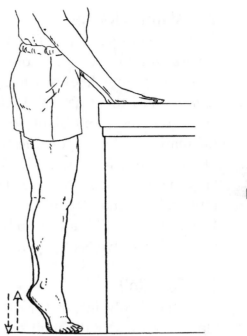

Ankle and Foot Exercises

Do these exercises sitting in a straight-backed chair with your feet bare. Have a bath towel and 10 marbles next to you. These exercises are for flexibility, strength, and comfort. This is a good time to examine your feet and toes for any signs of circulation or skin problems, and check your nails to see if they need trimming.

23. Towel Grabber

Spread a towel out in front of your chair. Place your feet on the towel, with your heels near the edge closest to you. Keep your heels down and your foot slightly raised. Scoot the towel back underneath your feet, by pulling it with your toes. When you have done as much as you can, reverse the toe motion and scoot the towel out again.

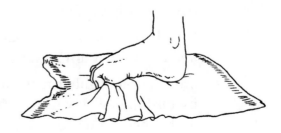

24. Marble Pick-Up

Do this exercise one foot at a time. Place several marbles on the floor between your feet. Keep your heel down, and pivot your toes toward the marbles. Pick up a marble with your toes, and pivot your foot to drop the marble as far as possible from where you picked it up. Repeat until all the marbles have been moved. Reverse the process and return all the marbles to the starting position. If marbles are difficult, try other objects, like jacks, dice, or wads of paper.

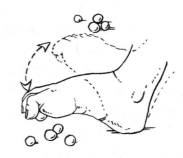

108

25. Foot Roll

Place a rolling pin (or a large dowel or closet rod) under the arch of your foot, and roll it back and forth. It feels great and stretches the ligaments in the arch of the foot.

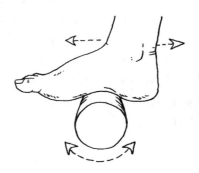

The Whole Body

26. The Stretcher

This exercise is a whole-body stretch to do lying on your back. Start the motion at your ankles as explained here, or reverse the process if you want to start with your arms first.

- Point your toes, and then pull your toes toward your nose. Relax.

- Bend your knees. Then flatten your knees and let them relax.

- Arch your back. Do the Pelvic Tilt. Relax.

- Breathe in, and stretch your arms above your head. Breathe out, and lower your arms. Relax.

- Stretch your right arm above your head, and stretch your left leg by pushing away with your heel. Hold for a count of 10. Switch to the other side and repeat.

Self-Tests

Whatever our goals, we all need to see that our efforts make a difference. Since an exercise program produces gradual change, it's often hard to tell if the program is working and to recognize improvement. Choose several of these flexibility and strength tests to measure your progress. Not everyone will be able to do all the tests. Choose those that work best for you. Perform each test before you start your exercise program, and record the results. After every four weeks, do the tests again and check your improvement.

1. Arm Flexibility

Do Exercise 6 (Pat and Reach) for both sides of the body. Ask someone to measure the distance between your fingertips.

Goal: Less distance between your fingertips.

2. Shoulder Flexibility

Stand facing a wall, with your toes touching the wall. One arm at a time, reach up the wall in front of you. Hold a pencil, or have someone mark how far you reached. Also do this sideways, standing about three inches (8 cm) away from the wall.

Goal: To reach higher.

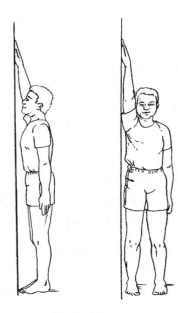

3. Hamstring Flexibility

Do the Hamstring Stretch (Exercise 20), one leg at a time. Keep your thigh perpendicular to your body. How much does your knee bend? How tight does the back of your leg feel?

Goal: Straighter knee and less tension in the back of the leg.

4. Ankle Flexibility

110

Sit in a chair with your bare feet flat on the floor and your knees bent at a 90-degree angle. Keep your heels on the floor. Raise your toes and the front of your foot. Ask someone to measure the distance between the ball of your foot and the floor.

Goal: One to two inches (3 to 5 cm) between your foot and the floor.

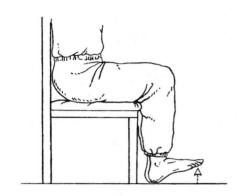

5. Abdominal Strength

Use the Curl-Up (Exercise 12). Count how many repetitions you can do before you get too tired to do more, or count how many you can do in one minute.

Goal: More repetitions.

6. Ankle Strength

This test has two parts. Stand at a table or counter for support.

- Do Exercise 22 (Tiptoes) as quickly and as often as you can. How many can you do before you tire?

- Stand with your feet flat. Put most of your weight on one foot, and quickly tap the floor with the front part of your other foot. How many taps can you do before you tire?

Goal: Ten to fifteen repetitions of each movement.

• • •

Suggested Further Reading

Cooper, Kenneth H. *The Aerobics Program for Total Well-Being: Exercise, Diet, Emotional Balance*. New York: Bantam Doubleday, 1985.

Nelson, Miriam E. *Strong Women Stay Young*. New York: Bantam Books, 1998.

Torkelson, Charlene. *Get Fit While You Sit: Easy Workout From Your Chair*. Berkeley, Calif.: Hunter House Publishing, 1999.

111

CHAPTER
8

Exercising for Endurance: Aerobic Activities

H OW MUCH IS ENOUGH? One of the biggest problems with endurance (aerobic) exercise is that it is easy to overdo, even for those who don't have a chronic illness. Inexperienced and misinformed exercisers think they have to work very hard for exercise to do any good. Exhaustion, sore muscles, painful joints, and shortness of breath are the results of jumping in too hard and too fast. As a result, some people may discontinue their exercise programs indefinitely, thinking that exercise is just not meant for them.

There is no magic formula for determining how much exercise you need. *The most important thing to remember is that some is better than none.* If you start slowly and increase your efforts gradually, it is likely that you will maintain your exercise program as a lifelong habit. Generally it is better to begin your conditioning program by underdoing rather than overdoing. Here are some rough guidelines to help you decide how much exercise is enough for you.

Several studies suggest that the *upper* limit of benefit is about 200 minutes of moderate-intensity aerobic exercise per week. Doing more than that doesn't gain you much (and it increases your risk of injury). On the other hand, doing 100 minutes of exercise per week gets you about 90% of the gain, while 60 minutes of aerobic exercise per week yields about 75% of the gain. Sixty minutes is just 15 minutes of mild aerobic exercise four times a week!

Let's take a closer look at some general guidelines for the frequency, duration, and intensity of aerobic exercise.

- *Frequency:* Three or four times a week is a good choice for aerobic exercise. Taking every other day off gives your body a chance to rest and recover. We recommend that you rest at least one day per week.

- *Time:* Start with just a few minutes, and gradually increase the duration of your aerobic activity to about 30 minutes a session. You can safely increase the time by alternating intervals of brisk exercise with intervals of rest or easy exercise. For example, after 3–5 minutes of brisk walking, do 1–2 minutes of easy strolling, then another 3–5 minutes of brisk walking. Eventually, you can build up to 30 minutes of activity. Then gradually eliminate rest intervals until you can maintain 20–30 minutes of brisk exercise. If 30 minutes seems too long, consider two sessions of 10–15 minutes each. Either way appears to improve health significantly.

- *Intensity:* Safe and effective endurance exercise should be done at no more than *moderate intensity*. High-intensity exercise increases the risk of injury and causes discomfort, so not many people stick with it. Exercise intensity is measured by how hard you work. For a trained runner, completing a mile in 12 minutes is probably low-intensity exercise. For a person who hasn't exercised in a long time, a brisk 10-minute walk may be of moderate to high intensity. For others with severe physical limitations, 1 minute may be of moderate intensity. The trick, of course, is to figure out what is moderate intensity for you. There are several easy ways to do this.

Talk Test

Talk to another person or yourself, sing, or recite poems out loud while you exercise. Moderate-intensity exercise allows you to speak comfortably. If you can't carry on a conversation or sing because you are breathing too hard or are short of breath, you're working too hard. Slow down. The talk test is an easy way to regulate exercise intensity.

If you have lung disease, the talk test might not work for you. If that is the case, try the perceived-exertion test.

Perceived Exertion

Another way to monitor intensity is to rate how hard you're working on a scale of 0 to 10. Zero, at the low end of the scale, is lying down, doing no work at all. Ten is equivalent to working as hard as possible, very hard work that you couldn't do longer than a few seconds. Of course, you never want to exercise that hard. A good level for your aerobic exercise routine is between 3 and 6 on this scale. At this level, you'll usually feel warmer, that you're breathing more deeply and faster than usual, that your heart is beating faster than normal, but you should not be feeling pain.

Remember, these are just rough guidelines on frequency, duration, and intensity, not a rigid prescription. Listen to your own body. Sometimes you need to tell yourself (and maybe others) that enough is enough. More exercise is not necessarily better, especially if it gives you more pain or discomfort. As *The Walking Magazine* said, "Go for the smiles, not the miles."

Heart Rate

Unless you're taking heart-regulating medication (such as the beta-blocker propranolol), monitoring your heart rate while exercising is one way to measure exercise intensity. The faster the heart beats, the harder you're working. (Your heart also beats fast when you are frightened or nervous, but here we're talking about how your heart responds to physical activity.) Endurance exercise at moderate intensity raises your heart rate into a range between 60 and 80 percent of your safe maximum heart rate. Safe maximum heart rate declines with age, so your safe exercise heart rate gets lower as you get older. You can follow the general guidelines of Table 8.1, "Age–Exercise Heart Rate," or calculate your individual exercise heart rate. Either way, you need to know how to take your pulse.

Take your pulse by placing the tips of your middle three fingers at your wrist below the base of your thumb. Feel around in that spot until you feel the pulsations of blood pumping with each heartbeat. Count how many beats you feel in 15 seconds. Multiply this number by 4 to find out how fast your heart is beating in one minute. Start by taking your pulse whenever you think of it, and you'll soon learn the difference between your resting and exercise heart rates.

How to calculate your own exercise heart rate range:
1. Subtract your age from 220:
   Example: 220 – 60 = 160   You: 220 – _____ = _____
2. To find the *lower end* of your exercise heart rate range, multiply your answer in step 1 by [.6]:
   Example: 160 × .6 = 96   You: _____ × .6 = _____
3. To find the *upper end* of your exercise heart rate range, which you *should not exceed,* multiply your answer in step 1 by [.8]:
   Example: 160 × .8 = 128   You: _____ × .8 = _____

Table 8.1 *Age–Exercise Heart Rate*

Age Range	Exercise Pulse (15 sec)
0–30	29–39
30–40	28–37
40–50	26–35
50–60	25–33
60–70	23–31
70–80	22–29
80+	16–24

116

The exercise heart rate range in our example is from 96 to 128 beats per minute. What is yours?

Most people count their pulse for 15 seconds, not a whole minute. To find your 15-second pulse, divide both the lower-end and upper-end numbers by 4. The person in our example should be able to count between 24 (96 ÷ 4) and 32 (128 ÷ 4) beats in 15 seconds while exercising.

The most important reason for knowing your exercise heart rate range is so that you can learn not to exercise too vigorously. After you've done your warm-up and 5 minutes of endurance exercise, take your pulse. If it's *higher than the upper rate, don't panic*. Slow down a bit. Don't work so hard.

At first, some people have trouble keeping their heart rate within the "ideal" heart rate range. Don't worry about that. Keep exercising at the level with which you're most comfortable. As you get more experienced and stronger, you will gradually be able to do more vigorous exercise while keeping your heart rate within your "goal" range. But don't let the target heart rate monitoring become a burden. Recent studies have shown that even low-intensity exercise can provide significant health benefits. So use the "ideal" heart rate range as a rough guide, but don't worry if you can't reach the lower end of that range. The important thing is to keep exercising!

If you are taking medicine that regulates your heart rate, have trouble feeling your pulse, or think that keeping track of your heart rate is a bother, use one of the other methods to monitor your exercise intensity.

How Much Is Enough? The FIT Formula

The results of your aerobic exercise program depend on how often you exercise (F = Frequency), how hard you work (I = Intensity), and how long you exercise each day (T = Time). In much the same way a doctor prescribes medicine to have a certain effect, you can select your own "exercise dose" to get the result you want. Your exercise dose comes from how you combine the frequency, intensity, and time of your exercise. A bigger dose gives you different benefits than a smaller dose.

117

- *Frequency:* Three to five days a week. Three days a week is the starting minimum. As you gain endurance and strength, you can do aerobic exercise more often. If you exercise more vigorously, 3 days is enough. If your aerobic exercise is a comfortably paced walk, you could build up to 5 or even 7 days a week.
- *Intensity:* No more than moderate intensity. Moderate intensity is being able to carry on a conversation while you exercise, a perceived-exertion level of no more than 6, or an exercise heart rate of no more than 75% of your age-predicted maximum heart rate.
- *Time:* Minimum of 30 minutes accumulated low to moderate physical activity. For health benefits, the activity may be accumulated in three 10-minute bouts during the day. To improve cardiovascular fitness, it may be necessary to exercise a bit longer each time.

People who are beginning an exercise program should consider following the recommendation in the *U.S. Surgeon General's Report on Physical Activity:* **Adults should accumulate 30 minutes of moderate physical activity on most days of the week.** It is important to remember that this is a goal, not necessarily your starting point. If you can begin exercising just 2 minutes at a time, you are likely to be able to reach the recommendation of 10 minutes three times a day and achieve important health benefits.

When to Warm Up and Cool Down

Warm-Up

If you are going to exercise at an intensity that causes you to breathe harder or your heart to beat faster, it is important to warm up first. A warm-up means that you do at least 5 minutes of a low-intensity activity to allow your heart, lungs, and circulation to gradually increase their work. If you are going for a brisk walk, warm up with 5 minutes of slow walking first. If you are riding a stationary bike, warm up with 5 minutes of no resistance and no more than 60 rpm (revolutions per minute). In an aerobic exercise class, you will warm up with a gentle routine before getting more vigorous. Warming up reduces the risk of injuries, soreness, and irregular heartbeats.

Cool Down

A cool-down period is important if you have exercised at an intensity that required you to breathe harder and your heart to beat faster, or if you felt warmer or perspired. Repeating the 5-minute warm-up activity or taking a slow walk helps your muscles gradually relax and your heart and breathing to slow down. Gentle stretching and flexibility exercises during the cool-down can be effective for increasing motion because your muscles and joints are warm and more easily stretched. Also, stretching gently now helps reduce the muscle soreness and stiffness that may follow vigorous exercise.

Endurance (Aerobic) Exercises

Many activities can be aerobic. We will examine in more detail a few of the more common ones, including walking, swimming, stationary bicycling, and low-impact aerobics.

Walking

Walking can condition your heart and lungs, strengthen bones and muscles, relieve tension, control weight, and generally make you feel good. Walking is easy, inexpensive, safe, and accessible. You can walk by yourself or with company, and you can take your exercise with you wherever you go. Walking is safer and puts less stress on the body than jogging or running. It's an especially good choice if you are older, have been sedentary, or have joint problems.

Most people with a chronic illness can walk as a fitness exercise. If you walk to shop, visit friends, and do household chores, then you'll probably be able to walk for exercise. Using a cane or walker need not stop you from getting into a walking routine. If you are in a wheelchair, use crutches, or experience more than mild discomfort when you walk a short distance, you should consider some other type of aerobic exercise, or consult a physician or therapist for help.

Be cautious the first two weeks of walking. If you haven't been doing much for a while, 10 minutes of walking may be enough. Build up your time with intervals of strolling. Each week increase the brisk walking interval by no more than 5 minutes until you are up to 20 or 30 minutes. Follow the frequency, duration, and intensity guidelines, and read these tips on walking before you start.

Walking Tips

Choose your ground. Walk on a flat, level surface. Walking on hills, uneven ground, soft earth, sand, or gravel is hard work and often leads to hip, knee, or foot pain. Fitness trails, shopping malls, school tracks, streets with sidewalks, and quiet neighborhoods are good places to get started.

Always warm up and cool down with a stroll. It's important to walk slowly for 3 to 5 minutes to prepare your circulation and muscles for a brisk walk, and to finish up with the same slow walk to let your body slow down gradually. Experienced walkers know they can avoid shin and foot discomfort when they begin and end with a stroll.

Set your own pace. It takes practice to find the right walking speed. To find your speed, start walking slowly for a few minutes, then increase your speed to a pace that is slightly faster than normal for you. After 5 minutes, monitor your exercise intensity by checking your pulse, or using the perceived-exertion or talk methods. If you are above the range or feel out of breath, slow down. If you are below the range, try walking a little faster. Walk another 5 minutes and check your intensity again. If you are still below your exercise range, keep walking at a comfortable speed and simply check your intensity in the middle and at the end of each walk.

Increase your arm work. You can also raise your heart rate into the "ideal" or target exercise range by increasing arm work. (Remember that many people with lung disease may want to avoid arm exercises, since they can cause more shortness of breath than other exercises.) Bend your elbows a bit and swing your arms more vigorously. Alternatively, carry a one- or two-pound weight (.75 kg) in each hand. You can purchase hand weights for walking, hold a can of food in each hand, or put sand, dried beans, or pennies in two small plastic beverage bottles or socks. The extra work you do with your arms increases your intensity of exercise without forcing you to walk faster than you find comfortable.

Shoes

It's not necessary to spend a lot of money on shoes. Wear shoes of the correct length and width with shock-absorbing soles and insoles. Make sure they're big enough in the toe area: The "rule of thumb" is a thumb width between the end of your longest toe and the end of the shoe. You shouldn't feel pressure on the sides or tops of your toes. The heel counter should hold your heel firmly in the shoe when you walk.

Wear shoes with a continuous crepe or composite sole in good repair. Shoes with leather soles and a separate heel don't absorb shock as well as the newer athletic and casual shoes. Shoes with laces or Velcro let you adjust width as needed and give more support than slip-ons. If you have problems tying laces, consider Velcro closures or elastic shoelaces.

120

Many people like shoes with removable insoles that can be exchanged for more-shock-absorbing ones. Insoles are available in sporting goods stores and shoe stores. When you shop for insoles, take your walking shoes with you. Try on the shoe with the insole to make sure that there's still enough room inside for your foot to be comfortable. Insoles come in sizes and can be trimmed with scissors for a final fit. If your toes take up extra room, try the three-quarter insoles that stop just short of your toes. If you have prescribed inserts in your shoes already, ask your doctor about insoles.

Possible Problems

If you have *pain around your shins* when you walk, you may not be spending enough time warming up. Try some ankle exercises before you start walking. Start your walk at a slow pace for at least 5 minutes. Keep your feet and toes relaxed.

Another common problem is *sore knees*. Fast walking puts stress on knee joints. To slow your speed and keep your heart rate up, try doing more work with your arms (see above). Do the Knee Strengthener and Ready-Go (Chapter 7, Exercises 17 and 19) in your warm-up to reduce knee pain.

Cramps in the calf and *heel pain* can be helped by doing the Achilles Stretch (Chapter 7, Exercise 21) before and after walking. A slow walk to warm up is also helpful. If you have circulatory problems in your legs, and experience cramps or pain in your calves while walking, alternate intervals of brisk and slow walking at whatever pace you can tolerate. Slow down and give your circulation a chance to catch up before the pain is so intense you have to stop. As you will see, such exercises may even help you to gradually walk farther with less cramping or pain. If this doesn't help, check with your physician or therapist for suggestions.

Maintain good posture. Remember the heads-up position in Chapter 7 and keep your shoulders relaxed to help reduce *neck and upper back discomfort*.

Swimming

Swimming is another good endurance exercise. The buoyancy of the water lets you move your joints through their full range of motion and strengthen your muscles and cardiovascular system with less stress than on land. Since swimming involves the arms, it can lead to excessive shortness of breath in people with lung disease. However, for people with asthma, swimming may be the preferred exercise as the moisture helps reduce shortness of breath. People with heart disease who have severely irregular heartbeats and have had an implantable "defibrillator" (AICD) permanently placed on their heart should avoid swimming. For most people with chronic illness, however, swimming is excellent exercise. It uses the whole body. If you haven't been swimming for a while, consider a refresher course.

To make swimming an endurance exercise, you will eventually need to swim continuously for 20 minutes. Use the frequency, duration, and intensity guidelines set out at the beginning of this chapter to build up your endurance. Try different strokes, modifying them or changing strokes after each lap or two. This lets you exercise all joints and muscles without overtiring any one area.

Swimming Tips

The breast stroke and crawl normally require a lot of neck motion and may be uncomfortable if you have neck pain. To solve this problem, use a *mask and snorkel* so that you can breathe without twisting your neck.

Chlorine can be irritating to eyes. Consider a good pair of *goggles*. You can even have swim goggles made in your eyeglass prescription.

A *hot shower* or soak in a hot tub after your workout helps reduce stiffness and muscle soreness. Remember not to work too hard or get too tired. If you're sore for more than two hours, go easier next time.

Always swim where there are qualified lifeguards if possible, or with a friend. Never swim alone.

Aquacize

If you don't like to swim, or are uncomfortable learning strokes, you can walk laps in the pool or join the millions who are "aquacizing"—exercising in water.

Aquacize is comfortable, fun, and effective as a flexibility, strengthening, and aerobic activity. The buoyancy of the water takes weight off hips, knees, feet, and back. Because of this, exercise in water is generally better tolerated than walking in people who have pain in the hips, knees, feet, and back. Exercising in a pool allows you a degree of privacy in doing your own routine, since no one can see you much below shoulder level.

Getting Started

Joining a water exercise class with a good instructor is an excellent way to get started. The Arthritis Foundation sponsors water exercise classes and trains instructors to teach them. The heart and lung associations can refer you to exercise programs that include aquacize classes. Contact your local chapter or branch office to see what is available. Many community and private health centers also offer water exercise classes, with some geared to older adults.

If you have access to a pool and want to exercise on your own, there are many water-exercise books available. One we recommend is *Hydrorobics*, by Joseph A. Krasevec and Diane C. Grimes (Human Kinetics Publishers, 1985). It contains a lot of good ideas for exercise in the water.

122

Water temperature is always a topic when people talk about water exercise. The Arthritis Foundation recommends a pool temperature of 84°F (29°C), with the surrounding air temperature in the same range. Except in warm climates, this means a heated pool. If you're just starting to aquacize, find a pool with these temperatures. If you can exercise more vigorously and don't have a condition known as Raynaud's phenomenon or other cold sensitivity, you can probably aquacize in cooler water. Many pools where people swim laps are about 80–83°F (27–28°C). It feels quite cool when you first get in, but starting off with water walking, jogging, or another whole-body exercise helps you warm up quickly.

The deeper the water you stand in, the less stress there is on joints; however, water above mid-chest can make it hard to keep your balance. You can let the water cover more of your body just by spreading your legs apart or bending your knees a bit.

Aquacize Tips

Wear something on your feet to protect them from rough pool floors and to provide traction in the pool and on the deck. Choices vary from terry cloth slippers with rubber soles (they stretch in water, so buy a size smaller than your shoe size) to footgear especially designed for water exercise. Some styles have Velcro tape to make them easier to put on. Beach shoes with rubber soles and mesh tops also work well.

If you are sensitive to cold or have Raynaud's phenomenon, *wear a pair of disposable latex surgical gloves*. Boxes of gloves are available at most pharmacies. The water trapped and warmed inside the glove seems to insulate the hand. If your body gets cold in the water, wear a T-shirt and/or full-leg Lycra exercise tights for warmth.

If the pool does not have steps, and it is difficult for you to climb up and down a ladder, *suggest positioning a three-step kitchen stool* in the pool by the ladder rails. This is an inexpensive way to provide steps for easier entry and exit, and it is easy to remove and store when not needed.

Wearing a *flotation belt or life vest* adds extra buoyancy, to take weight off hips, knees, and feet. That makes exercising more comfortable for these joints.

You can *regulate how hard you work* in the water by the way you move. To make the work easier, move slowly. Another way to regulate exercise intensity is to change how much water you push when you move. For example, when you move your arms back and forth in front of you under water, it is hard work if you hold your palms facing each other and clap. It is easier if you turn your palms down and slice your arms back and forth with only the narrow edge of your hands pushing against the water.

If you have asthma, exercising in water helps to avoid the worsening of asthma symptoms that occur during other types of exercise. This is probably due to the beneficial effect of water vapor on the lungs. Remember, though, that for many people with lung disease, exercises involving the arms can cause more shortness of breath than leg exercises. You may want to focus most of your aquacizing, therefore, on exercises involving mainly the legs.

If you have had a stroke, or have another condition that may affect your strength and balance, make sure that you have someone to help you in and out of the pool. Finding a position close to the wall or staying close to a buddy who can lend a hand if needed are ways to add to your safety and security. You may even wish to sit on a chair in fairly shallow water as you do water exercises. Ask the instructor to help you design the best exercise program, equipment, and facilities for your specific needs.

Stationary Bicycling

Stationary bicycles offer the fitness benefits of bicycling without the outdoor hazards. They're preferable for people who don't have the flexibility, strength, or balance to be comfortable pedaling and steering on the road. Some people with paralysis of one of their legs or arms can exercise on stationary bicycles with special attachments for their paralyzed limb. Indoor use of stationary bicycles may also be preferable to outdoor bicycling for people who live in a cold or hilly area.

The stationary bicycle is a particularly *good alternative exercise*. It doesn't put excess strain on your hips, knees, and feet, you can easily adjust how hard you work, and weather doesn't matter. Use the bicycle on days when you don't want to walk or do more vigorous exercise, or can't exercise outside.

Make it Interesting

The most common complaint about riding a stationary bike is that it's boring. If you ride while watching television, reading, or listening to music, you can

---

Stationary-Bicycle Checklist

❏ The bicycle is steady when you get on and off. The resistance is easy to set and can be set to zero. The seat is comfortable.

❏ The seat can be adjusted for full knee extension when the pedal is at its lowest point.

❏ Large pedals and loose pedal straps allow feet to move slightly while pedaling.

❏ There is ample clearance from the frame for knees and ankles.

❏ The handlebars allow good posture and comfortable arm position.

---

become fit without becoming bored. One woman keeps interested by mapping out tours of places she would like to visit and then charts her progress on the map as she rolls off the miles. Other people set their bicycle time for the half hour of soap opera or news that they watch every day. There are videocassettes of exotic bike tours that put you in the rider's perspective. Book racks that clip on to the handlebars make reading easy.

Riding Tips

Bicycling uses different muscles than walking. Until your leg muscles get used to pedaling, you may be able to ride only a few minutes. Start off with no resistance. Increase resistance slightly every two weeks. Increasing resistance has the same effect as bicycling up hills. If you use too much resistance, your knees are likely to hurt, and you'll have to stop too soon before you get the benefit of endurance.

Pedal at a comfortable speed. For most people, 50–60 revolutions per minute (rpm) is a good place to start. Some bicycles tell you the rpm, or you can count the number of times your right foot reaches its lowest point in a minute. As you get used to bicycling, you can increase your speed. However, faster is not necessarily better. Listening to music at the right tempo makes it easier to pedal at a consistent speed. Experience will tell you the best combination of speed and resistance.

Set your goal for *20 to 30 minutes of pedaling* at a comfortable speed. Build up your time by alternating intervals of brisk pedaling with less exertion. Use your heart rate, perceived exertion, or the talk test to make sure you aren't working too hard. If you're alone, try singing songs as you pedal. If you get out of breath, slow down.

Keep a record of the times and distances of your "bike trips." You'll be amazed at how much you can do.

On bad days, keep your exercise habit going by pedaling with no resistance, at fewer rpm, or for a shorter period of time.

Other Exercise Equipment

125

If you have trouble getting on or off a stationary bicycle, or don't have room for a bicycle where you live, you might try a restorator or arm crank. Ask your therapist or doctor, or call a medical supply house.

A *restorator* is a small piece of equipment with foot pedals which can be attached to the foot of a bed or placed on the floor in front of a chair. It allows you to exercise by pedaling. Resistance can be varied, and placement of the restorator lets you adjust for leg length and knee bend. A restorator can be a good alternative to an exercise bicycle for people who have problems with balance, weakness, or paralysis. People with other chronic illnesses, such as lung disease, may find the restorator to be an enjoyable first step in getting an exercise program started.

Arm cranks are bicycles for the arms. They are mounted on a table. People who are unable to use their legs for active exercise can improve their cardiovascular fitness and upper-body strength by using the arm crank. It's important to work closely with a therapist to set up your program, because using only your arms for endurance exercise requires different intensity monitoring than using the bigger leg muscles. As mentioned previously, many people with lung disease may find arm exercises to be less enjoyable than leg exercises since they may experience shortness of breath.

There is a wide variety of exercise equipment in addition to what we've mentioned so far. These include treadmills, self-powered and motor-driven rowing machines, cross-country skiing machines, mini-trampolines, and stair-climbing machines. Most are available in both commercial and home models. If you're thinking about exercise equipment, have your objectives clearly in mind. For cardiovascular fitness and endurance, you want equipment that will help you exercise as much of your body at one time as possible. The motion should be rhythmical, repetitive, and continuous. The equipment should be comfortable, safe, and not stressful on joints. If you're interested in a new piece of equipment, try it out for a week or two before buying it.

Exercise equipment that requires you to use *weights* usually does not improve cardiovascular fitness unless individualized "circuit training" can be designed. A weight-lifting program alone builds strength, but it can put excessive stress on joints, muscles, tendons, and ligaments. Most people will find that the flexibility and strengthening exercises in this book will help them safely achieve significant increases in strength as well as flexibility. Be sure that you consult with your doctor or therapist if you prefer to add strengthening exercises involving weights or weight machines to your program.

Low-Impact Aerobics

Most people find *low-impact aerobic dance* a fun and safe form of exercise. "Low impact" means that one foot is always on the floor and there is no jumping. However, low impact does not necessarily mean low intensity, nor do the low-impact routines protect all joints. If you participate in a low-impact aerobic class, you'll probably need to make some modifications based on your condition.

Getting Started

Start off by *letting the instructor know who you are,* that you may modify some movements to meet your needs, and that you may need to ask for advice. It's easier to start off with a newly formed class than it is to join an ongoing class. If you don't know people, try to get acquainted. Be open about why you may sometimes do things a little differently. You'll be more comfortable and may find others who also have special needs.

Most instructors use music or count to a specific beat and do a set number of repetitions. You may find that the movement is too fast or that you don't want to do as many repetitions. *Modify the routine* by slowing down to half-time, or keep up with the beat until you start to tire and then slow down or stop. If the class is doing an exercise that involves arms and legs and you get tired, try resting your arms and do only the leg movements, or just walk in place until you are ready to go again. Most instructors will be able to instruct you in "chair aerobics" if you need some time off your feet.

Some low-impact routines use a lot of *arm movements* done at or above shoulder level to raise heart rates. Remember that for people with lung disease, hypertension, or shoulder problems, too much arm exercise above shoulder level can worsen shortness of breath, increase blood pressure, or cause pain, respectively. Modify the exercise by lowering your arms or taking a rest break.

Being different from the group in a room walled with mirrors takes courage, conviction, and a sense of humor. The most important thing you can do for yourself is to *choose an instructor who encourages everyone to exercise at her or his own pace* and a class where people are friendly and having fun. Observe classes, speak with instructors, and participate in at least one class session before making any financial commitment.

Aerobic Studio Tips

Wear shoes. Many studios have cushioned floors and soft carpet that might tempt you to go barefoot. Don't! Shoes help protect the small joints and muscles in your feet and ankles by providing a firm, flat surface on which to stand.

Protect your knees. Stand with knees straight but relaxed. Many low-impact routines are done with bent, tensed knees and a lot of bobbing up and down. This can be painful and is unnecessarily stressful. Avoid this by remembering to keep your knees relaxed (aerobics instructors call this "soft" knees). Watch in the mirror to see that you keep the top of your head steady as you exercise. Don't bob up and down.

Don't overstretch. The beginning (warm-up) and end (cool-down) of the session will have stretching and strengthening exercises. Remember to stretch only as far as you comfortably can. Hold the position and don't bounce. If the stretch hurts, don't do it. Ask your instructor for a less stressful substitute, or choose one of your own.

Change movements. Do this often enough so that you don't get sore muscles or joints. It's normal to feel some new sensations in your muscles and around your joints when you start a new exercise program. However, if you feel discomfort doing the same movement for some time, change movements or stop for a while and rest.

Alternate kinds of exercise. Many exercise facilities have a variety of exercise opportunities: equipment rooms with cardiovascular machines, pools, and aerobic studios. If you have trouble with an hour-long aerobic class, see if you can join the class for the warm-up and cool-down and use a stationary bicycle or treadmill for your aerobic portion. Many people have found that this routine gives them the benefits of both an individualized program and group exercise.

Self-Tests for Endurance/Aerobic Fitness

For some people, just the feelings of increased endurance and well-being are enough to demonstrate progress. Others may find it helpful to demonstrate that their exercise program is making a measurable difference. You may wish to try one or both of these endurance/aerobic fitness tests before you start your exercise program.

Not everyone will be able to do both tests, so pick one that works best for you. Record your results. After four weeks of exercise, do the test again and check your improvement. Measure yourself again after four more weeks.

Distance Test

Find a place to walk, bicycle, swim, or water-walk where you can measure distance. A running track works well. On a street you can measure distance with a car. A stationary bicycle with an odometer provides the equivalent measurement. If you plan on swimming or water walking, you can count lengths of the pool.

After a warm-up, note your starting point and bicycle, or swim, or walk as briskly as you *comfortably* can for 5 minutes. Try to move at a steady pace for the full time. At the end of 5 minutes, mark your spot or note the distance or laps and immediately take your pulse and rate your perceived exertion from 0 to 10. Continue at a slow pace for 3 to 5 more minutes to cool down. Record the distance, your heart rate, and your perceived exertion.

Repeat the test after several weeks of exercise. There may be a change in as soon as four weeks. However, it often takes eight to twelve weeks to see improvement.

Goal: To cover more distance *or* to lower your heart rate *or* to lower your perceived exertion.

Time Test

Measure a given distance to walk, bike, swim, or water-walk. Estimate how far you think you can go in 1 to 5 minutes. You can pick a number of blocks, actual distance, or lengths in a pool.

Spend 3 to 5 minutes warming up. Start timing and start moving steadily, briskly, and comfortably. At the finish, record how long it took you to cover your course, your heart rate, and your perceived exertion.

Repeat after several weeks of exercise. You may see changes in as soon as four weeks. However, it often takes eight to twelve weeks for a noticeable improvement.

Goal: To complete the course in less time *or* at a lower heart rate *or* at a lower perceived exertion.

• • •

Suggested Further Reading

Stewart, Gordon W. *Active Living: The Miracle of Medicine for a Long and Healthy Life.* Champaign, Ill.: Human Kinetics Publishers, 1995.

Weddington, Michael. *Aerobic Sports Log: A Revolutionary Graphical Log Book for the Health-Conscious Individual.* Griffin Publishing,1997.

CHAPTER
9

Exercising Tips for People with Specific Chronic Illnesses

U NTIL NOW, OUR SUGGESTIONS HAVE BEEN APPLICABLE to nearly everyone with a chronic illness. Here are some specific recommendations to help you answer any questions you may still have about exercise and your particular chronic health problem.

Heart Disease

If you have heart disease, you probably have had one or more of the following conditions:

1. Myocardial infarction (heart attack)
2. Coronary bypass surgery
3. Coronary "balloon" angioplasty
4. Angina pectoris (chest pain or discomfort)

It is important for you to understand, however, that exercise can be both safe and beneficial for many people who have experienced these conditions. It is also important for you to work closely with your doctor to design an exercise program that is safe and beneficial for you. Remember that exercise has been shown to not only improve the quality of one's life but also may improve the quantity of one's life. Following are some general exercise guidelines for people with heart disease.

Should I Limit My Exercise Because of My Heart Disease?

Restrictions on conditioning activities may be necessary for some people with heart disease because of one or more of three conditions:

1. Evidence of an ongoing restriction to blood flow to the heart muscle *(ischemia)*.
2. Presence of frequent and dangerous irregular heartbeats *(arrhythmias)*.
3. *Decreased pumping strength* of the heart muscle.

132

Your doctor will be able to tell you if you have any of these conditions by examining you and performing tests such as an electrocardiogram (EKG), exercise treadmill test, echocardiogram, or coronary angiogram (see Chapter 16).

If you do *not* have any of the above conditions, it is safe for you to begin the conditioning program outlined in this book, with common sense as your only restriction. For example, common sense would tell you that you shouldn't try to run a marathon during your first week of conditioning.

One word of caution: Strengthening activities, such as *weight lifting* or *rowing,* are generally quite safe but can lead to increased blood pressure, especially for those people with preexisting high blood pressure. Straining (holding your breath as you lift or row) can put unnecessary stress on the heart. If you and your doctor think weight lifting should be part of your conditioning program, remember to breathe out as you are lifting. One way of being sure to breathe is to sing or talk while you are exercising.

If you have any of the three conditions (ischemia, arrhythmias, or decreased pumping strength in the heart muscle), your doctor may wish to place one or more of the following restrictions on your activity:

Begin your conditioning program in a supervised setting, such as a cardiac rehabilitation program at your local hospital or community center. Even those people with heart disease who don't have any of the three conditions listed above may prefer the supervision and structure of a rehabilitation program.

Once you are cleared for activity by your physician, *always keep the intensity of your activity well below the intensity that produces symptoms,* such as chest pain or severe shortness of breath. For example, if you get chest pain during an exercise treadmill test when your heart is beating at 130 beats per minute, you should never let your heart get above 115 beats per minute. Some people can easily judge the intensity of their activity so that it always stays below their "danger zone," but other people find it difficult to do so. For them, it may be easier to wear a pulse rate monitor (available at most medical supply stores) so that they can see their heart rate as they exercise. If you prefer, remember that you can monitor the intensity of your exercise by two other methods—the talk test and your perceived exertion (see page 114).

If your heart disease is severe enough, your doctor may want to change your treatment before giving you clearance to exercise. For example, if you have severely limited blood flow to the heart muscle, your doctor may want to treat you with a medicine that suppresses the arrhythmias, or may want to either treat you with special medicines or recommend that you have bypass surgery or "balloon" angioplasty to improve the blood flow to the heart muscle before clearing you for conditioning activities.

Activities that cause you to strain, such as weight lifting and rowing, may be harmful for people whose hearts have decreased pumping strength and should be avoided. Safer and more beneficial conditioning activities include light calisthenics, walking, swimming, and stationary bicycling.

Exercising in the recumbent position (lying down)—such as when you swim or pedal a special "recumbent" stationary bicycle—can help improve the efficiency of the heart's pumping action, except for people with severely damaged hearts (those who have had "heart failure," for example). You may or may not find such exercise to be less taxing for you.

Finally, always remember that if you develop new or different symptoms, such as chest pain, shortness of breath, or rapid or irregular heartbeats while at rest or while exercising, you should temporarily discontinue your conditioning activities and contact your physician.

Lung Disease

Exercise training has been found to increase endurance, reduce symptoms, and reduce hospital visits for people with chronic lung disease. Remember that your exercise routine should begin at a very low intensity. Gradually begin to increase your activity, moving from short bouts of exercise to relatively longer ones. With time you'll notice that the shortness of breath at a given level of exertion will start to decrease. Work with your doctor to plan the safest, most beneficial exercise program for you. A few important points to remember:

Use your medicine, particularly your inhaler, *before you exercise.* It will help you exercise longer and with less shortness of breath.

If you become severely short of breath with only minimal exertion, your doctor may want to change your medicines, or even have you use supplemental oxygen before you begin your conditioning activities.

Take plenty of time to warm up and cool down during conditioning activities. This should include exercises such as pursed-lip breathing and diaphragmatic, or abdominal, breathing (see page 44). The best exercise is probably a daily routine of low intensity, which you can add to gradually. Remember that when exercising, mild shortness of breath is normal. Remember also that before you begin to exercise you will experience a normal "anticipatory" increase in your heart rate and breathing rate. This is normal, but can be intimidating and fatiguing for some people. This makes it even more important to follow a gradual warm-up routine that includes pursed-lip breathing techniques. Be sure to avoid your "trouble zones" of shortness of breath by keeping the duration and intensity of your exercise well below those levels causing severe shortness of breath.

Concentrate on your breathing, making sure you breathe in deeply and slowly. Use pursed-lip breathing when you breathe out (see page 44). Practice so that you take two or three times as much time breathing out as you do breathing in. For example, if you are walking briskly and notice that you can take 2 steps while you're breathing in, you should breathe out through pursed lips over 4 to 6 steps. Breathing out slowly will help you exchange air in your lungs better and will probably increase your endurance.

Remember that *arm exercises may cause shortness of breath sooner* than leg exercises.

Likewise, *cold and dry air can make breathing and exercise more difficult.* This is why swimming is an especially good activity for people with chronic lung disease.

Strengthening exercises such as calisthenics, light weight lifting, and rowing *may be helpful,* particularly for people who have become weakened or deconditioned from medications, such as steroids.

Using a restorator (see page 125) is especially appropriate for some people with lung disease who have a low level of endurance or are fearful of exerting themselves. The restorator allows a person to remain seated and to start and stop at their pleasure. It's a good device to build confidence and get accustomed to exertion in a secure atmosphere.

A Special Note for Those with Severe Lung Disease

Many people with severe lung disease believe that it is impossible to exercise. Getting across a room may take a great deal of effort. If this sounds like you, exercise is especially important. Here are some tips:

Move slowly. When crossing a room or going to the bathroom, many people with lung disease hurry up to get there before their breath runs out. It is much better to slow down. Move slowly, breathing as you go. At first, this will take a real effort, as the tendency is to speed up. With a little practice, you will find that you can go farther with less effort. If you are afraid to try this alone, have someone walk with you, carrying a chair (a folding "cane chair" might be useful), so that you can sit down if needed. Remember, slow and steady is always better. *Don't forget to breathe as you walk.*

Everyone with lung disease who can get out of bed can exercise 10 minutes a day. Here is how you do it. Every hour, get up from what you are doing and **walk slowly** across the room or around your chair **for 1 minute**. Doing this 10 times a day will give you your 10 minutes of exercise.

After you have done this for a week or two and are feeling a little stronger, then walk 2 minutes every hour. You have just doubled your exercise and are now up to 20 minutes a day. When this feels comfortable (in another week or two), change your pattern to walking 3–4 minutes every other hour. Again, wait a week or two and try 5 minutes 3 or 4 times a day. Next, try 6–7 minutes 2 or 3 times a day. You now have the basic idea. Most people with severe lung disease can build up to walking 10 to 20 minutes, once or twice a day, within a couple of months.

The rules are the same as for any other exercise:

1. Start with what you can do now. A minute an hour is great!
2. Add to your program very gradually, every week to two.
3. If you ever feel worse after you finish than before you started, cut back on the amount of time you exercise.
4. Move slowly.
5. Remember to breathe while exercising.

Stroke

Physical activity, especially physical therapy, is a cornerstone in the recovery of a person with stroke. Strengthening and flexibility exercises help people regain the use of arms and legs that have been affected. Before beginning the conditioning program described in preceding chapters, *check with your doctor to make sure your blood pressure is under control.* (See the section on hypertension, on page 136.)

If you have weakness or poor balance from your stroke, some activities may cause you to *strain, lose your balance, or fall.* It may be wise to use a walker, cane, or stick with a partner while you are exercising. You may also wish to sit or alternate sitting and standing during your conditioning, especially if you have weakness in your legs. You may find a restorator helpful with your program. If an arm is affected, you may prefer to do leg exercises. If both a leg and arm are

135

affected, it is probably best to begin with seated exercise. Remember that while a conditioning program can increase your strength, vigor, and endurance, it may not bring improvement to a severely weakened or paralyzed limb. If you have a prescribed exercise program already, talk with your therapist for ideas to combine your therapeutic exercise with a conditioning exercise program.

Claudication

Exercise for people with claudication in their legs is generally limited only by the leg pain that develops during exercise. The good news is that conditioning exercises can help improve endurance and reduce leg pain for most people. The bad news is that people with claudication sometimes find it impossible to do any type of leg exercises, thus keeping them from getting the benefit of a conditioning program. In this case, they usually need to have bypass surgery on the vessels in their affected leg.

To gradually improve endurance and lessen leg pain, *daily short periods* of leg exercise (walking, bicycling, etc.) should be performed *just short of the point of leg pain.* When the discomfort starts, rest, slow down, or change activities until it subsides. Then the short period of exercise should be repeated, again to the point of some discomfort, but not severe pain. This *cycle of exercise and rest* should initially be repeated for 5–10 minutes and, with time, gradually increased to 30–60 minutes. Many people find that they can gradually increase the length of time they can walk comfortably or exercise with this method. Remember, arm exercises won't usually cause leg pain, so be sure to include them as an important part of your conditioning program.

Other methods that may help delay calf pain when you walk are to wear "rocker-bottom" shoes or to walk more slowly and use more arm swing.

Hypertension

Before beginning a conditioning program, a person with high blood pressure should *check with a doctor to make sure that his or her blood pressure is under control.* This generally means that it consistently runs somewhere around 160/90 or less. The first blood pressure number (160) is the systolic blood pressure. This part of the blood pressure reading will normally go up during vigorous exercise, but for someone with hypertension it should never be allowed to go above 200. The second blood pressure reading is the diastolic blood pressure, which generally does not increase during exercise.

You should avoid exercises that can potentially worsen your hypertension, such as those causing you to strain while holding your breath (isometrics, weight lifting, and rowing, for example). Also, exercising with arms overhead will cause increased blood pressure and heart rate and should be avoided. Include endurance exercises that rhythmically contract and relax muscles in your program. These are generally not harmful, but can actually be of benefit because they help lower both your blood pressure and your weight.

To be safe, you may want to monitor your own blood pressure at the beginning, middle, and end of your exercise time as you begin to establish your program. (Blood pressure monitors can be purchased in most pharmacies and are generally easy to use. Instructions are provided, of course.) If your blood pressure is ever higher than 200/110, temporarily discontinue your conditioning exercises until you speak with your physician about the need for possible changes in your hypertension treatment plan.

Osteoarthritis

Since osteoarthritis begins as primarily a problem with joint cartilage, an exercise program should include taking care of cartilage. *Cartilage needs joint motion and some weight bearing to stay healthy.* In much the same way that a sponge soaks up and squeezes out water, joint cartilage soaks up nutrients and fluid and gets rid of waste products by being squeezed when you move the joint. If the joint is not moved regularly, cartilage deteriorates. If the joint is continually compressed, as the hips and knees are by long periods of standing, the cartilage can't expand and soak up nutrients and fluid.

Any joint with osteoarthritis should be *moved through its full range of motion several times daily* to maintain flexibility and to take care of the cartilage. Judge your activity level so pain is not increased. If hips and knees are involved, walking and standing should be limited to no more than two to four hours at a time, followed by at least an hour off your feet to give the cartilage time to decompress. Using a cane on the opposite side of the painful hip or knee will reduce joint stress and often get you over a rough time. Good posture, strong muscles and good endurance, as well as shoes that absorb the shocks of walking, are important ways to protect cartilage and reduce joint pain. Knee strengthening exercises (Exercises 17, 18, and 19) performed daily can help reduce knee pain and protect the joint.

Osteoporosis

Regular exercise plays an important part in preventing osteoporosis and strengthening bones already showing signs of disease. *Endurance and strengthening exercises* are the most effective for *strengthening bone*. Flexibility and back and abdominal strengthening exercises are important for *maintaining good posture*. Look for the VIP exercises in Chapter 7. You can help yourself with a regular exercise program that includes some walking and general flexibility and strengthening of your back and stomach muscles.

If you have osteoporosis, or think that you may be at risk for this condition, here are some exercise precautions to remember:

- *No heavy lifting.*
- *Avoid falls.* Be careful on pool decks, waxed floors, icy sidewalks, or cluttered surfaces.
- *Don't bend down to touch your toes when standing.* This puts unnecessary pressure on your back. If you want to stretch your legs or back, lie on your back and bring your knees up toward your chest.
- *Sit up straight, and don't slouch.* Good sitting posture puts less pressure on the back.
- *If your balance is poor* or you feel clumsy, consider using a cane or walking stick when you're in a crowd or on unfamiliar ground.

Rheumatoid Arthritis

People with rheumatoid arthritis should pay special attention to *flexibility, strengthening, and appropriate use of their joints.* Maintaining good posture and joint motion will help joints, ease pain, and avoid tightness. Arthritis pain and long periods spent sitting or lying down can quickly lead to poor posture and limited motion, even in the joints not affected by arthritis. Be sure to include hand and wrist exercises in your daily program. A good time to do these is after washing dishes or during a bath when hands are warm and limber.

Rheumatoid arthritis sometimes affects the bones in the neck. It is best to *avoid extreme neck movements* and not to put pressure on the back of the neck or head.

Stiffness in the morning can be a big problem. Flexibility exercises before getting up or during a hot bath or shower seem to help. A favorite way to get loosened up is to "stretch like a cat and then shake like a dog." Also, doing gentle flexibility exercises in the evening before bed have been shown to reduce morning stiffness.

Diabetes

Regular exercises can be an important part of controlling blood glucose levels and improving health for everyone with diabetes. However, people who are taking medication to control diabetes should discuss any change in exercise habits with their doctor or nutritionist because changes in activity levels often require changes in medication and eating schedules.

Exercise is beneficial for people with diabetes in several ways. Mild to moderate aerobic exercise decreases the need for insulin and helps control blood glucose levels by increasing the sensitivity of body cells to insulin and lowering blood glucose levels both during and after exercise. This type of regular exercise also is essential for losing weight and reducing cardiovascular risk factors such as high blood lipid levels and high blood pressure.

The exercise program recommended for people with diabetes is generally the same as the conditioning program described earlier. Mild to moderate aerobic exercise for no more than 40 minutes performed as part of a general conditioning program in the morning or early afternoon is a safe and effective way to help control diabetes and stay healthy.

Additional considerations for exercise with diabetes are to begin an exercise program only when your diabetes is under good control, keep in touch with your doctor to make changes in medication and diet if needed, and coordinate eating, medication, and exercise to avoid hypoglycemia. If you have problems with sensation or poor circulation, be sure to check skin regularly and protect yourself from blisters and abrasions. It is especially important to inspect your feet and practice good skin and nail hygiene regularly. Shoe inserts can be made to help protect the soles of the feet.

• • •

Suggested Further Reading

Cooper, Kenneth H. *Overcoming Hypertension: Dr. Kenneth Cooper's Preventative Medicine Program.* New York: Bantam, 1991.

Sayce, Valerie, and Ian Fraser. *Exercise Beats Arthritis: An Easy-to-Follow Program of Exercises.* Palo Alto, Calif.: Bull Publishing, 1998, and Melbourne, Australia: Fraser Publications, 1987.

Van Fulpen, Diane C. *Guide to Contented Hearts: Cardiac Risk Management: Cholesterol, High Blood Pressure, Exercise, Stress, Weight, Diet.* Contented Hearts, Inc., 1995.

Vedral, Joyce L. *Bone Building and Body Shaping Workout.* New York: Simon and Schuster, 1998.

White, Martha. *Water Exercise: 78 Safe and Effective Exercises for Fitness and Therapy.* Champaign, Ill.: Human Kinetics Publishers, 1995.

CHAPTER
10
Communicating

141

"**Y**OU JUST DON'T UNDERSTAND!"" How often has this statement, expressed or unexpressed, summed up a frustrating verbal exchange? The goal in any communication between people is first that the other person understands what you are trying to say. Feeling you are not understood leads to frustration, and a prolonged feeling of frustration can lead to depression, anger, and helplessness. These are not good feelings for anyone, especially people with chronic illness. Dealing with a chronic illness can be frustrating enough, without adding communication problems.

Poor communication is the biggest factor in poor relationships, whether they be between spouses, other family members or friends, coworkers, or doctors and patients. Even in casual relationships, poor communication causes frustration. How often have you been angry and frustrated as a customer, and how often is this because of poor communication?

When you have a chronic illness, good communication becomes a necessity. Your health care team, in particular, *must* "understand" you. As a self-manager, it is in your best interest to learn the skills necessary to make your communications as effective as possible.

In this chapter, we discuss ways to improve the communication process. Specifically, these are ways to express feelings in a positive way, how to ask for help, how to say "no," as well as how to best listen and how to get more information from the other person.

While reading this chapter, keep in mind that *communication is a two-way street.* As uncomfortable as you may feel about expressing your feelings and asking for help, chances are that others are also feeling this way. It may be up to you to make sure the lines of communication are open. Be careful not to get caught in being uncomfortable with others because "they should know . . . ."

Expressing Your Feelings

Having a chronic condition brings about many feelings, some of them not pleasant. Here are some hints on how to express these feelings in a positive and constructive manner.

Start by taking a few moments to review exactly what is the situation that is bothering you and what you are feelng. For example, John and Steve had agreed to go together to a sporting event. When John came to pick up Steve, he was not ready and was not sure he wanted to go as he was having some trouble with his arthritic knees. The following conversation took place.

John: Why do you always spoil my plans? At least you could have called and I could have asked my son to go with me.

Steve: You just don't understand. If you had pain like I do, you wouldn't be so quick to criticize. You don't think of anyone but yourself.

John: Well, I can see that I should just go by myself.

In the above situation, neither John nor Steve had stopped to think about what was really bothering them or how they felt about it. Rather, they both blamed the other for an unfortunate situation.

The following is the same conversation in which both people were using thoughtful communications.

John: When we have made plans and then at the last minute you are not sure you can go, I feel frustrated and angry. I don't know what to do—go on without you, stay here and change our plans, or just not make future plans.

Steve: When this arthritis acts up at the last minute, I am also confused. I keep hoping I can go and so don't call you because I don't want to disappoint you and I really want to go. I keep hoping that my knees will get better as the day wears on.

John: I understand.

Steve: Let's go to the game. You can let me off at the gate before parking so I won't have to walk as far. Then I can do the steps slowly and be in our seats when you arrive. I do want us to keep making plans. In the future, I will let you know sooner if I think my arthritis as acting up.

John: Sounds good to me. I really do like your company and also knowing how I can help. It is just that being caught by surprise makes me angry.

John and Steve talked about the specific situation and how they felt about it. Neither blamed the other. Unfortunately, we are often in situations where the other person is using blaming communications or we are caught not listening and reverting to blaming communications. Even in this situation, thoughtful communication can be helpful. Look at the following example.

Jan: Why do you always spoil my plans? At least you could have called. I am really tired of trying to do anything with you.

Sandra: I understand. When this asthma acts up at the last minute, I am confused. I keep hoping I can go and so don't call you because I don't want to disappoint you and I really want to go. I keep hoping that I will get better as the day wears on.

Jan: Well, I hope that in the future you will call. I don't like being caught by surprise.

Sandra: I understand. If it is OK with you, let's go shopping now. I can walk a short way and rest in the coffee shop with my book while you continue to shop. I do want us to keep making plans. In the future, I will let you know sooner if I think my asthma is acting up.

In this last example, only Sandra is using thoughtful communication. Jan continues to blame. The outcome, however, is still positive with both people accomplishing what they want. The following are some suggestions for accomplishing good communications.

1. Always show regard for the other person. Avoid demeaning or blaming comments such as when Jan says, "Why do you always spoil my plans?" The use of the word "you" is a clue that your communication might be blaming.

2. Be clear. Describe a specific situation. For example, Sandra said, "When this asthma acts up at the last minute, I am confused. I keep hoping I can go and so don't call you because I don't want to disappoint you and I really want to go. I keep hoping that I will get better as the day wears on."

3. Test your assumptions verbally. Jan did not do this. She assumed that Sandra was being rude by not calling her. Remember that assumptions are often the place where good communications break down. One sign that you are making assumptions is when you are thinking "he or she should know . . . ."

144

4. Be open and honest about your feelings. Sandra did this when she talked about wanting to go, not wanting to disappoint Jan, and hoping that her asthma would get better.

5. Accept the feelings of others and try to understand them. This is not always easy. Sometimes you need to think about what has been said. Rather than answer immediately, remember that it is always acceptable to use "I understand" or "I don't fully understand. Could you explain some more?"

6. Be tactful and courteous. You can do this by avoiding sarcasm and blaming.

7. Work at using humor, but at the same time know when to be serious.

8. Be careful not to make yourself a victim by not expressing your needs and feelings and then expecting others to act the way you think they "should" act.

9. Finally, become a good listener.

"I" Messages

Many of us are uncomfortable expressing our feelings. This discomfort can be acute if doing so means we might seem critical of the person we're talking to.

Especially if emotions are high, attempts to express frustration can be laden with *"you" messages* that suggest blame. Its direction is toward the other person, causing the other person to feel as though he or she is under attack. Suddenly, the other person feels on the defensive, and protective barriers go up. The person trying to express feelings, in turn, feels greater anxiety when faced with these defensive barriers and the situation escalates to anger, frustration, and bad feelings.

The use of "I," however, doesn't strike out or blame. It is another form of communication that helps to express how *you* feel, rather than how the other person makes you feel. Here are some examples of *"I" messages:*

"You" message:	Why are *you* always late? We never get anywhere on time.
"I" message:	*I* get really upset when *I'm* late. It's important to *me* to be on time.
"You" message:	There's no way *you* can understand how lousy I feel.
"I" message:	*I'm* not feeling well. *I* could really use a little help today.

145

Watch out for *hidden* "you" messages. These are "you" messages with *"I feel . . ."* stuck in front of them. Here's an example:

"You" message:	*You* always walk too fast.
HIDDEN *"You" message:*	*I feel* angry when *you* walk so fast.
"I" message:	*I* have a hard time walking fast.

The trick to "I" messages is to avoid the use of the word *you,* and, instead, report your personal feelings using the word *I.* Of course, like any new skill, "I" messages take practice. Start by really listening, both to yourself and to others. Take some of the "you" messages you hear and turn them into "I" messages in your head. By playing this word game in your head, you'll be surprised at how fast they become a habit in your own expressions.

There are some cautions to note when using "I" messages. First, they are not panaceas. Sometimes the listener has to have time to hear them. This is especially true if "you" messages and blaming have been the more usual ways of communicating. Even if at first using "I" messages seems ineffective, continue to use them and refine your skill.

Exercise—"I" Messages

Change the following statements into "I" messages. (Watch out for "hidden you" messages!)

You expect me to wait on you hand and foot!

Doctor, you never have enough time for me. You're always in a hurry.

You hardly ever touch me anymore. You haven't paid any attention to me since my heart attack.

You didn't tell me the side effects of all these drugs you're giving me or why I have to take them, doctor.

146

Also, some people may use "I" messages as a means of manipulation. If used in this way, problems can escalate. To be used effectively, "I" messages must report *honest* feelings.

One last note: "I" messages are an excellent way to express *positive* feelings and compliments! *"I* really appreciate the extra time you gave me today, doctor."

Asking for Help

Problems with communication around the subject of help are pretty common. For some reason, many people feel awkward about asking for help or in refusing help. Although this is probably a universal problem, it can come up more often for people with chronic illness.

It may be emotionally difficult for some of us to ask for needed help. Maybe it's difficult for us to admit to ourselves that we are unable to do things as easily as in the past. When this is the case, try to avoid hedging your request: "I'm sorry to have to ask this . . ." "I know this is asking a lot . . ." "I hate to ask this, but . . ." Hedging tends to put the other person on the defensive: "Gosh, what's he going to ask for that's so much, anyway?" Be specific about what help you are requesting. A general request can lead to misunderstanding, and the person can react negatively to insufficient information.

General request:	I know this is the last thing you want to do, but I need help moving. Will you help me?
Reaction:	Uh . . . well . . . I don't know. Um . . . can I get back to you after I check my schedule? [probably next year!]
Specific request:	I'm moving next week, and I'd like to move my books and kitchen stuff ahead of time. Would you mind helping me load and unload the boxes in my car Saturday morning? I think it can be done in one trip.
Reaction:	I'm busy Saturday morning, but I could give you a hand Friday night, if you'd like.

People with chronic illness also sometimes deal with offers of help that are not needed or desired. In most cases, these offers come from people who are dear to you and genuinely want to be helpful. A well-worded "I" message can refuse the help tactfully, without embarrassing the other person. "Thank you for being so thoughtful, but today I think I can handle it myself. I'd like to be able to take you up on your offer another time, though."

Saying "No"

Suppose, however, you are the one being asked to help someone. Responding readily with "yes" or "no" may not be advisable. Often, we need more information before we can respond to the request.

If the request lacks enough information for us to respond, often our first feelings are negative. The example we just discussed about helping a person move is a good one. "Help me move" can mean anything from moving furniture up stairs to picking up the pizza for the hungry troops. Again, using skills that get at the specifics will aid the communication process. It is important to understand what the *specific* request is before responding. *Asking for more information or paraphrasing* the request will often help clarify the request, especially if prefaced by a phrase such as "Before I answer . . . " (this will hopefully prevent the person whose request you are paraphrasing from thinking that you are going to say yes).

Once you know what the specific request is and have decided to decline, it is important to *acknowledge the importance of the request* to the other person. In this way, the person will see that you are rejecting the *request,* rather than the *person.* Your turn-down should not be a put-down. "You know, that's a worthwhile project you're doing, but I think it's beyond my capabilities this week." Again, specifics are the key. Try to be clear about the conditions of your turn-down: Will you always turn down this request, or is it just that today or this week or right now is a problem?

148

Listening

This is probably the most important communication skill. Most of us are much better at talking than we are at listening. We need to actually listen to what the other person is *saying and feeling.* Most of us are already preparing a response, instead of just listening. There are several levels involved in being a good listener.

1. *Listen to the words and tone of voice, and observe body language.* Sometimes it is difficult to begin a conversation if there is a problem. There may be times when the words being used don't tell you there is something bothering this person. Is the voice wavering? Does he or she appear to be struggling to find "the right words"? Do you notice body tension? Does he or she seem distracted? If you pick up on some of these signs, this person probably has more on her or his mind than words are expressing.

2. *Acknowledge having heard the other person.* Let the person know you heard them. This may be a simple "uh huh." Many times the only thing the other person wants is acknowledgment, or just someone to listen, because sometimes merely talking to a sympathetic listener is helpful.

3. *Acknowledge the content of the problem.* Let the other person know you heard both the content and emotional level of the problem. You can do this by restating the content of what you heard. For example: "You are planning a trip." Or you can respond by acknowledging the emotions: "That must be difficult," or "How sad you must feel." When you respond on an emotional level, the results are often startling. These responses tend to open the gates for more expression of feelings and thoughts. Responding to either the content or emotion can help communication along by discouraging the other person from simply repeating what has been said.

4. *Respond by seeking more information.* (See next section.) This is especially important if you are not completely clear about what is being said or what is wanted. There is more than one useful method for seeking and getting information.

Getting More Information

Getting more information from another person is a bit of an art, requiring special consideration. It can involve techniques that may be simple, or more subtle.

Ask for more. This is the simplest way to get more information. "Tell me more" will probably get you more, as will "I don't understand . . . please explain," "I would like to know more about . . . ," "Would you say that another way?" "How do you mean?" "I'm not sure I got that," and "Could you expand on that?"

Paraphrase. This is a good tool if you want to make sure you understand what the other person meant (not just what he/she *said,* but *meant*). Paraphrasing can either help or hinder effective communication, depending on the way the paraphrase is worded, though. It is important to remember to paraphrase in the form of a question, not a statement. For example, assume another person says:

> *Well, I don't know. I'm really not feeling up to par. This party will be crowded, there'll probably be smokers there, and I really don't know the hosts very well, anyway.*

If we were to paraphrase this as a *statement* rather than a question, it might look like this:

> *Obviously, you're telling me you don't want to go to the party.*

Paraphrased as a *question:*

> *Are you saying that you'd rather stay home than go to the party?*

The response to the first paraphrase might be anger:

> *No, I didn't say that! If you're going to be that way, I'll stay home for sure.*

Or the response might be no response . . . a total shutdown of the communication, because of either anger or despair ("He just doesn't understand."). People don't like to be told what they meant.

149

On the other hand, the response to the second paraphrase might be

That's not what I meant. I'm just feeling a little nervous about meeting new people. I'd appreciate it if you'd stay near me during the party. I'd feel better about it, and I might have a good time.

As you can see, the second paraphrase promotes further communication, and you have discovered the real reason the person was expressing doubt about the party. You have gotten more information from the second paraphrase and no new information from the first one.

150

Be specific. If you want specific information, you must ask specific questions. We often automatically speak in generalities. For example:

Doctor: How have you been feeling?   *Patient:*   Not so good.

The doctor doesn't have much in the way of information about the patient's condition. "Not good" isn't very useful. Here's how the doctor gets more information:

Doctor: Are you still having those sharp pains in your left arm?   *Patient:*   Yes. A lot.

Doctor: How often?   *Patient:*   A couple of times a day.

Doctor: How long do they last?   *Patient:*   A long time.

Doctor: About how many minutes, would you say?

. . . and so on.

Physicians have been trained in ways to get specific information from patients, but most of us have not been trained to ask specific questions. Again, simply *asking for specifics* often works: "Can you be more specific about . . .?" "Are you thinking of something particular?" If you want to know "why," be specific about what it is. If you ask a specific question, you will be more likely to get a specific answer.

Simply asking *"Why?"* can unnecessarily prolong your attempt to get specific information. In addition to being a general rather than a specific word, "why" also makes a person think in terms of cause and effect, and he or she may respond at an entirely different level than you had in mind.

Most of us have had the experience where a three-year-old just keeps asking "Why?" over and over and over again, until the information the child wants is finally obtained (or the parent runs from the room, screaming). The poor parent doesn't have the faintest idea what the child has in mind and answers "Because . . ." in an increasingly specific order until the child's question is answered. Sometimes, however, the direction the answers take is entirely different than the child's question, and the child never gets the information he or she wanted. Rather than "why," begin your responses with "who," "which," "when," or "where." These words promote a specific response.

One last note about getting information: Sometimes we do not get the correct information because we do not know what question to ask. For example, you may be seeking legal services from a senior center. You call and ask if they have a lawyer and hang up when the answer is no. If, instead, you had asked where you might get low-cost legal advice, you may have gotten two or three referrals.

Communicating with Your Doctor

As a person with chronic illness, it is especially important to establish and maintain good communication with your doctor. The relationship you have with him/her must be looked on as a long-term one requiring regular work, much like a business partnership or a marriage.

Your doctor will probably know more intimate details about you than anyone except perhaps your spouse or your parents. You, in turn, should feel comfortable expressing your fears, asking questions that you may think are "stupid," and negotiating a treatment plan to satisfy you both, without feeling "put down" or that your doctor is not interested.

There are two things to keep in mind that will help to open, and keep open, the lines of communication with your doctor. How does the doctor feel? Too often, we expect our doctors to act as a warmhearted computer—a gigantic brain, stuffed with knowledge about the human body, and especially *your* human body, able to analyze the situation and produce a diagnosis, prognosis, and treatment on demand—*and* be a warm, caring person who makes you feel as though you're the only person he or she cares about taking care of.

Actually, most doctors wish they were just that sort of person, but no doctor can be all things to all patients. They are human, too. They get headaches, they get tired, and they get sore feet. They have families who demand their time and attention, and they have to fight bureaucracies as formidable as the rest of us face.

Most doctors entered the grueling medical training system because they wanted to make sick people well. It is frustrating for them not to be able to cure someone with a chronic disease like emphysema or arthritis. They must take their satisfaction from improvements rather than cures, or even in maintenance of existing conditions rather than declines. Undoubtedly, you have been frustrated, angry, or depressed from time to time about your illness, but bear in mind that your doctor has probably felt similar emotions about his or her inability to make you well. In this, you are truly partners.

Second, in this partnership between you and your doctor, *the biggest threat to a good relationship and good communication is **time***. If you or your doctor could have a fantasy about the best thing to happen in your relationship, it would probably involve more time for you both, more time to discuss things, more time to explain things, more time to explore options. When time is short, the anxiety it produces can bring about rushed messages, often "you" messages, and messages that are just plain misunderstood—with no time to correct them.

A doctor is usually on a very tight schedule. This fact becomes painfully obvious to you when you have had to wait in the doctor's office because of an emergency that has delayed your appointment. Doctors try to stay on schedule, and sometimes patients and doctors alike feel rushed as a consequence. One way to help you to get the most from your visit with the doctor is to take **P.A.R.T.**

152

| **Prepare** | **Ask** | **Repeat** | **Take action** |

Prepare

Before visiting or calling your doctor, *prepare your "agenda."* What are the reasons for your visit? What do you expect from your doctor?

Take some time to make a written list of your concerns or questions. But be realistic. If you have 13 different problems, it isn't likely that your doctor can adequately deal with that many concerns in one visit. Identify your main concerns or problems. Writing them down also helps you remember them. Have you ever thought to yourself, after you walked out of the doctor's office, "Why didn't I ask about . . . ?" or "I forgot to mention . . . ." Making a list beforehand helps you ensure your main concerns get addressed.

Mention your main concerns right at the beginning of the visit. Don't wait until the end of the appointment to bring up concerns, because there won't be the time to properly deal with them. Give your list to the doctor. If the list is long, expect that only two or three items will be addressed this visit, and let your doctor know which items are the most important to you. Studies show that doctors allow an average of 18 seconds for the patient to state his or her concerns before interrupting with focused questioning. Preparing your questions in advance will help you use your 18 seconds well.

As an example of bringing up your concerns at the beginning of the visit, when the doctor asks, "What brings you in today?" you might say something like "I have a lot of things I want to discuss this visit," *(looking at his or her watch and appointment schedule, the doctor immediately begins to feel anxious),* "but I know that we have a limited amount of time. The things that most concern me are my shoulder pain, my dizziness, and the side effects from one of the medications I'm taking," *(the doctor feels relieved because the concerns are focused and potentially manageable within the appointment time available).*

Try to be as open as you can in sharing your thoughts, feelings, and fears. Remember, your physician is not a mind reader. If you are worried, try to explain why: "I am worried that what I have may be contagious," or "My father had similar symptoms before he died," and so on. The more open you are, the more likely it is that your doctor can help you. If you have a problem, don't wait for the doctor to "discover" it. State your concern immediately. For example, "I am worried about this mole on my chest."

Give your physician feedback. If you don't like the way you have been treated by the physician or someone else on the health care team, let your physician know. If you were unable to follow the physician's advice or had problems with a treatment, tell your physician so that adjustments can be made. Also, most physicians appreciate compliments and positive feedback, but patients are often hesitant to praise their doctors. So, if you are pleased, remember to let your physician know it.

Preparing for a visit involves more than just listing your concerns. You should be prepared to *concisely describe your symptoms to the doctor* (when they started, how long they last, where they are located, what makes them better or worse, whether you have had similar problems before, whether you have changed your diet, exercise, or medications in a way that might contribute to the symptoms, etc.). If a treatment has been tried, you should be prepared to report the effect of the treatment. And if you have previous records or test results that might be relevant to your problems, bring them along. Be sure to tell your doctor about the trends (are you getting better or worse or are you the same?) and tempo (is it faster or slower?) of your problem, not just how you feel today. For example, "In general I am slowly getting better, although today I do not feel well." In treating a chronic condition, the trends and tempo are very important.

Ask

Another key to effective doctor-patient communication is asking questions. Getting understandable answers and information is one of the cornerstones of self-management. You need to be prepared to ask questions about diagnosis, tests, treatments, and follow-up.

1. *Diagnosis:* Ask your doctor what's wrong, what caused it, if it is contagious, what is the future outlook (or prognosis), and what can be done to prevent it in the future.

2. *Tests:* Ask your doctor if any medical tests are necessary, how they will affect your treatment, how accurate they are, and what is likely to happen if you are not tested. If you decide to have a test, find out how to prepare for the test and what it will be like.

3. *Treatments:* Ask about your treatment options including lifestyle change, medications, surgery. Inquire about the risks and benefits of treatment and the consequences of not treating.

4. *Follow-up:* Find out if and when you should call or return for a follow-up visit. What symptoms should you watch for, and what should you do if they occur?

You may wish to take some notes on important points during the visit or consider bringing along someone else to act as a second listener. Another set of eyes and ears may help you later recall some of the details of the visit or instruction.

Repeat

It is extremely helpful to briefly repeat back to the doctor some of the key points from the visit and discussion. These might include diagnosis, prognosis, next steps, treatment actions, and so on. This is to double-check that you clearly understood the most important information. Repeating back also gives the doctor a chance to quickly correct any misunderstandings and miscommunications. If you don't understand or remember something the physician said, admit that you need to go over it again. For example, you might say, "I'm pretty sure you told me some of this before, but I'm still confused about it." Don't be afraid too ask what you may consider a "stupid" question. These questions can often indicate an important concern or misunderstanding.

154

Take Action

When the visit is ending, you need to clearly understand what to do next. When appropriate, ask your physician to write down instructions or recommend reading material for more information on a particular subject.

If, for some reason, you can't or won't follow the doctor's advice, let the doctor know. For example, "I didn't take the aspirin. It gives me stomach problems," or "My insurance doesn't cover that much physical therapy, so I can't afford it," or "I've tried to exercise before, but I can't seem to keep it up." If your doctor knows why you can't or won't follow advice, alternative suggestions can sometimes be made to help you overcome the barrier. If you don't share the barriers to taking actions, it's difficult for your doctor to help.

Asking for a Second Opinion

Many people find it uncomfortable to ask their doctor for a second opinion about their diagnosis or treatment. Especially if you have a long relationship with your doctor or simply *like* him or her, patients sometimes worry that asking for another opinion might be interpreted by the doctor as questioning his or her competence. It is a rare doctor whose feelings will be hurt by a sincere request for another opinion. If your condition is medically complicated or difficult, the doctor may have already consulted with another doctor (or more) about your case, at least on an informal basis.

Even if your condition is not particularly complicated, asking for a second opinion is a perfectly acceptable, and often expected, request. Doctors prefer a straightforward request, and asking in a nonthreatening "I" message will make this task simple:

> I'm *still feeling confused and uncomfortable about this treatment.* I *feel another opinion might help* me *feel more reassured. Can you suggest someone I could consult?*

In this way, you have expressed your own feelings without suggesting that the doctor is at fault. You have also confirmed your confidence in him or her by asking that he or she suggest the other doctor. (Remember, however, that you are not bound by his or her suggestion; you may choose anyone you wish for a second opinion.)

Good communication skills help make life easier for everyone, especially when chronic illness enters the picture. The skills discussed in this chapter, though brief, will hopefully help smooth the communication process. In summary, the box on the next page gives examples of some words that can help or hinder.

155

Words That Help	Words That Hinder
Right now, at this time, at this point, today	Never, always, every time, constantly
I	You
Who, which, where, when	Obviously . . .
How do you mean, please explain, tell me more, I don't understand	Why

Working with the Health Care System

Today many of the frustrations we have with doctors are really frustrations with new systems of health care. We seem to have less and less time with our doctor and more and more time waiting. In many countries, health care has become big business with both the doctor and patient playing supporting roles. If you are frustrated because your waiting time is too long, it takes too long to get an appointment, you don't have enough time with the doctor, or you can't get the treatment or medication you need, your doctor probably has the same frustration.

If you are unhappy with your health care system, don't just steam—do something. Find out who is running the system and how decisions are made. Then make your feelings felt by letter, phone, or e-mail. Most health care systems want to keep you as a patient, and thus when they get pushed enough by patients, they usually respond. The problem is that the decision makers tend to isolate themselves, so it is much easier to make your feelings known to a receptionist, nurse, or doctor. These people have little or no power in the system. However, they can often tell you who to call or write. The more you can form a partnership with your physician, the more the two of you can make your health care system responsive.

• • •

Suggested Further Reading

Beach, Wayne A. *Conversation About Illness*. Lawrence Erlbaum, 1996.

Beck, Aaron. *Love Is Never Enough: How Couples Can Overcome Misunderstandings, Resolve Conflicts, and Solve Relationship Problems Through Cognitive Therapy*. New York: Harper Collins, 1989.

Golde, Robert A. *What You Say Is What You Get*. New York: Hawthorn Books, 1979.

Jones, J. Alfred, Gary L. Kreps, and Gerald M. Phillips. *Communicating with Your Doctor: Getting the Most out of Health Care*. Hampton Press, 1995.

McKay, Matthew, Martha Davis, and Patrick Fanning. *Messages: The Communication Skills Book*. Oakland, Calif.: New Harbinger Publications, 1983.

CHAPTER
11

Sex and Intimacy

COUPLES WHO LIVE WITH A CHRONIC HEALTH PROBLEM, with either one partner or both having a problem, face a challenge in keeping this important part of their relationship alive and well. Fear of injury or of bringing about a health emergency can dampen desire in one or both partners. Likewise, fear of increasing symptoms can frustrate couples, even if the symptoms occur only during sex itself. Sex, after all, is supposed to be joyful and pleasurable, not scary or uncomfortable!

For humans, sex is more than the act of sexual intercourse; it is also the sharing of physical and emotional sensuality. There is a special intimacy when we make love. Believe it or not, having a chronic health problem might actually improve your sex life by causing you to experiment with new types of physical and emotional stimulation for you and your partner. This process of exploring sensuality with your partner can open communication and strengthen your relationship, as well. Additionally, natural "feel-good" hormones, called "endorphins," are released in our bloodstreams when we have sex.

For many people with chronic conditions, it is intercourse itself that is most difficult to sustain, because of the physical demands it places on our bodies. Intercourse brings about increased heart rate and breathing and can tax someone with limited energy or breathing or circulatory problems. Therefore, it is helpful to spend more time on sensuality or foreplay and less on actual intercourse. By concentrating on ways to arouse your partner and give pleasure while in a comfortable position, your intimate time together can last longer and be very satisfying. Many people enjoy climax without intercourse; others may wish to climax with intercourse. For some, climax may not be as important as sharing pleasure and they are satisfied without an orgasm. No matter how or if climax is reached, uncomfortable symptoms can be minimized if we concentrate on foreplay and sensuality rather than intercourse itself. There are many ways to enhance sensuality during sexual activity. In sex, as in most things, our minds and bodies are linked. By recognizing this, we can increase the sexual pleasure we experience through both physical and cognitive stimulation.

Emotional concerns can also be a serious factor for someone with health problems. Someone who has had a heart attack or a stroke is often concerned that sexual activity will bring on another attack. People with breathing difficulties worry that sex is too strenuous and will bring on an attack of coughing and wheezing, or worse. Their partners may fear that sexual activity might cause these problems, or even death, and fear they would be responsible.

160

One of the most subtle and devastating barriers to fulfilling sexuality is the damage that has been caused to a person's self-image and self-esteem. Many report that they believe they are physically unattractive as a result of their disease—their paralysis, their shortness of breath, their weight gain from medications, or the changing shape of their joints—a sense of not being a whole, functioning being. This causes them to avoid sexual situations, and they "try not to think about it." This often leads to depression, and depression leads to lack of interest in sex, and that leads to depression . . . a vicious cycle. Depression can be treated and you can feel better. For more on depression and how to help yourself overcome it, see Chapter 4.

Even good sex can get better, though. Thankfully, there are ways you and your partner can explore sensuality and intimacy, as well as some ways to overcome fear during sex.

Overcoming Fear during Sex

Anyone who has experienced a chronic condition has experienced fear that it will get worse, or even that an episode could be life-threatening. Health problems can really get in the way of the activities that we want and need to do. When sex is the activity that fear affects, we have a difficult problem: Not only are we denying ourselves an important, pleasurable part of life, but we probably feel guilty about denying our partner the same. Our partner may even feel more fearful and guilty than we do—afraid that he or she might hurt us during sex and guilty for maybe feeling resentful. This dynamic can cause serious problems in a relationship, and the stress and depression these problems cause can even cause more symptoms. We don't have to allow this to happen!

Remember the real estate maxim: "The three most important things to consider when buying a house are location, location, and location"? Well, for successful sexual relationships, the three most important things are (1) communication, (2) communication, and (3) communication! The most effective way to address the fears of both partners is to confront them and find ways to alleviate them through effective communication and problem solving. Without effective communication, learning new positions and ways to increase sensuality are not going to be enough. This is particularly important for people who may worry about how their health problem may make them look physically to others. Often, they find that their partner is far less concerned than they are.

When you and your partner are comfortable with talking about sex, you can go about finding solutions to the problems your chronic health problem imposes on you. To start with, you can share what kinds of physical stimulation you prefer and which positions you find most comfortable. Then you can share the fantasies you find most arousing. It's difficult to dwell on fears when your mind is occupied with a fantasy!

To get this process started, you and your partner may find some help with communication skills in Chapter 10 and problem-solving techniques in Chapter 2. Remember, if these techniques are new, give them time and practice. As we find with any new skill, it takes patience to learn to do them well.

Sensuality with Touch

The largest sensual organ of our bodies is the skin. It is rich with sensory nerves. The right touch on almost any area of our skin can be very erotic. Fortunately, sexual stimulation through touch can be done in just about any position. It can be further enhanced with the use of oils, flavored lotions, feathers, fur gloves—turn your imagination loose on this one! Just about any part of the skin can be an erogenous zone, but the most popular are the mouth (of course!), ear lobes, neck, breasts (for both genders), navel area, hands (fingertips if you are giving pleasure, palms if you are receiving pleasure), wrists, small of the back, buttocks, toes, and insides of the thighs and arms. Experiment with the type of touch—some find a light touch arousing, others prefer a firm touch. It is not necessary to limit yourself to your hands, either. Many people become very aroused when touched with the lips, tongue, or sex toys.

Sensuality with Fantasy

What goes on in our minds can be extremely arousing. If it weren't, there would be no strip clubs, pornography, or even romance novels. Most people engage in sexual fantasy at some time or another. There are probably as many sex-

161

ual fantasies as there are people, and any are OK to mentally indulge in. If you discover a fantasy you and your partner share, you can play it out in bed, even if it is as simple as a particular saying you or your partner like to hear during sex. Engaging the mind during sexual activity can be every bit as arousing as the physical stimulation. It is also useful when symptoms during sex interfere with your enjoyment.

Overcoming Symptoms during Sex

162

Some people are unable to find a sexual position that is completely comfortable, or they find pain, shortness of breath, or fatigue during sex to be so distracting that it interferes with their enjoyment of sex or their ability to have an orgasm. This situation can pose some special problems. If you are unable to climax, you may feel resentful of your partner if he or she is able to climax, and your partner may feel guilty about it. If you avoid sex because you are frustrated, your partner may become resentful and you may feel guilty. Your self-esteem may suffer. Your relationship with your partner may suffer. Everything suffers.

One thing you can do to help deal with this situation is to time taking medication to be at peak effectiveness when you want to have sex. Of course, this would involve planning ahead! The type of medication may be important, too. If you take a narcotic-type pain reliever, for example, or one containing muscle relaxants or tranquilizers, you may find that your sensory nerves are dulled along with your pain. Obviously, it would be counterproductive to dull the nerves that will give you pleasure. Your thinking may also be muddled due to the medication and make it more difficult to focus. Some medications can also make it difficult for a man to achieve an erection. Ask your doctor or pharmacist about possible timing or alternatives if this is a problem for you.

Another way to deal with uncomfortable symptoms is to become the world's best expert at fantasy! To be really good at something, you have to train for it, and this is no exception. The idea here is to develop one or more sexual fantasies that you can indulge in when needed, making it vivid in your mind. Then, during sex, you can call up your fantasy and concentrate on it. By concentrating on the fantasy, or on picturing you and your partner making love while you actually are, you are keeping your mind consumed with erotic thoughts rather than your symptoms. However, if you have not had experience in visualization and imagery techniques, generally used for relaxation exercises such as those in Chapter 5, you will need to practice several times a week to learn it well. All of this practice need not be on your chosen sexual fantasy, however. You can start with any guided imagery tape or script such as the one in Chapter 5, working to make it more vivid each time you practice. Start with just picturing the images. When you get good at that, add and dwell on colors; then, in your mind, look down to your feet as you walk; then listen to the sounds around you; then concentrate on the smells and tastes in the image and feel your skin being touched by a breeze or mist; and, finally, feel yourself touch things in the image. Work on one of the senses at a time. Become good at one before going on to another. Once proficient at imagery, you can invest your own sexual fantasy and picture it, hear it, smell it, and feel it. You can even begin your fantasy by picturing yourself setting your symptoms aside. The possibilities are limited only by your imagination!

Learning to call on this level of concentration can also help you focus on the moment. Really focusing on your physical and emotional sensations during sex can be powerfully erotic. If your mind wanders (this is normal), gently bring it back to the here and now. ***IMPORTANT:*** *Do not try to overcome chest pain in this way. Chest pain should not be ignored, and a physician should be consulted right away.*

If you decide that you wish to abstain from sexual activity because of your chronic health problem, or if it is not an important part of your life, that's OK—but it is important to your relationship with your partner that he or she be in agreement with your decision. Good communication skills are essential in this situation, and you may even benefit from both of you discussing the situation with a professional therapist present. Someone trained to deal with important interpersonal situations can help facilitate the discussion.

Sexual Positions

In order to minimize symptoms during sex, as well as to minimize fear of pain or injury for both partners, it is important to find positions that are comfortable for both partners. Generally, comfortable positions can be found through experimentation. Everybody is different; no one position is good for everyone. We encourage you to experiment with different positions, possibly before you and your partner are too aroused for you to want to change to a more comfortable position. Experiment with placement of pillows or with using a sitting position on a chair.

No matter which position you try, it is often helpful to do some warm-up exercises before sex. Look at some of the stretching exercises from Chapter 7. Exercise can help your sex life in other ways, as well. Becoming more fit is an excellent way to increase comfort and endurance during sex. Walking, swimming, bicycling, and so on, can benefit you in bed as well as anywhere else by reducing

163

shortness of breath, fatigue, and pain. Also, learn your limits and pace yourself, just as you would with any other physical activity.

During sexual activity, it may be advisable to change positions periodically if your symptoms come on or increase when you stay in one position too long. This can also be done in a playful fashion, whereby it becomes fun for both of you instead of a chore. Stopping to rest is OK!

Special Considerations

164

There are specific issues that are of concern for people with certain health problems. People who are recovering from a heart attack or stroke, for example, are often afraid to resume sexual relations for fear of not being able to perform or of bringing on another attack or even death. It is even more common for their partners to refrain because of this fear. Fortunately, this is a myth, and sexual relations can be resumed as soon as you feel ready to do so. With stroke, in particular, there may be residual paralysis or weakness requiring a little more attention to finding the best positions for support and comfort and the most sensitive areas of the body to caress. There may also be concerns about bowel and bladder control that require consideration. The American Heart Association (www.americanheart.org) has some excellent guides to sexuality for those with heart disease and stroke, as well as information about Viagra and its risks for men with erection problems.

People with diabetes sometimes report problems with sexual function. Men may have difficulty achieving or maintaining an erection, which can be caused by medication side effects or other medical conditions associated with diabetes. Women and men can have reduced feeling (neuropathy) in the genital area. Women's most common complaint is inadequate vaginal lubrication. For people with diabetes, the most effective ways to prevent or lessen these problems is to maintain tight control of blood sugar, exercise, keep a positive outlook, and generally take care of themselves. Lubricants can help with sensitivity for both men and women. If you are using condoms, be sure to use a water-based lubricant. Petroleum-based lubricants destroy latex. The use of a vibrator can be very helpful for those with neuropathy, and concentrating on the most sensual parts of the body for stimulation can help make sex pleasurable. There are new therapies for men with erectile problems. The American Diabetes Association (www.diabetes.org) has more detailed information about sex and diabetes.

Chronic or recurring pain can put a big damper on sexual interest. It can be difficult to feel sexy when you hurt or are afraid that sex will make you hurt. People with pain as the predominant symptom of arthritis, migraine headaches, bowel disease, or the like, often have the challenge of having to overcome pain in order to become sexually aroused or to have an orgasm. This is one area where concentration and focus as discussed earlier in this chapter are most helpful skills. Learning to focus on the moment or on sexual fantasy can distract you away from the pain and allow you to concentrate on sex and your partner. Take your pain medication to have maximum effect during sex, find a comfortable position, take it slow and easy, relax, and enjoy extended foreplay. The Arthritis Foundation (www.arthritis.org) offers suggestions of positions for those with joint or back pain.

No matter what your chronic health problem, your doctor should be your first consultant about solutions to sexual problems caused by your condition. Sometimes something as simple as changing medication or its timing can make a difference. It's unlikely that your problem is unique—your doctor has probably heard about it before and may have some solutions to offer. Remember, this is just another problem associated with your chronic condition, just like fatigue, pain, and physical limitations, and it is a problem that can be addressed. Chronic health problems need not end sex. Through good communication and planning, satisfying sex can prevail. By being creative and willing to experiment, both the sex and the relationship involved can actually be better.

● ● ●

Suggested Further Reading

Carlton, Lucille. *In Sickness and in Health: Sex, Love and Chronic Illness*. Miami, Fla.: National Parkinson Foundation, Inc., 1996.

Klein, Marty. *Ask Me Anything: A Sex Therapist Answers the Most Important Questions for the 90's*. Pacifica Press, 1996.

Ornstein, Robert, and David Sobel. *Healthy Pleasures*. Reading, Mass.: Addison-Wesley, Longman Inc., 1990.

Robbins, Riki, and Marty Klein. *Let Me Count the Ways: Discovering Sex Without Intercourse*. New York: J. P. Tarcher, 1999.

Sandowski, Carol L. *Sexual Concerns When Illness or Disability Strikes*. Springfield, Ill.: Charles C. Thomas Publisher Ltd., 1990.

Seidman, David. *The Longevity Sourcebook*. Los Angeles: Lowell House, 1997.

CHAPTER
12

Making Your Wishes Known:
Advance Directives for Health Care

167

I

T HAS BEEN SAID THAT LIFE IS THE GREATEST RISK FACTOR FOR DYING. All of us have feelings about our own death. Death may be feared, welcomed, accepted, or, all too often, pushed aside to be thought about at a different time. Somewhere, in the back of our minds, most of us have ideas about how and when we would like to die. For some of us, life is so important that we feel everything should be done to sustain it. For others, life is important only so long as we can be active participants. For many people, the issue isn't really death but, rather, dying. We have all heard about the eighty-year-old who died skiing. This may be considered a "good" death. On the other hand, we may have a friend or family member who spent years in a nursing home unaware of his or her surroundings. This is usually not what we would wish for ourselves.

While none of us can have absolute control over our own deaths, this, like the rest of our lives, is something we can help manage. That is, we can have input, make decisions, and probably add a great deal to the quality of our death. Proper management can lessen the negative impacts of our death on our survivors. This chapter deals with information to help you manage better some of the legal issues of death, specifically advance directives for health care, usually known in the United States as durable powers of attorney for health care. While each state has different regulations, this information should be useful wherever you live. To get information and forms specific for your state, write: Choice In Dying, 475 Riverside Dr., New York, NY 10015, 1-800-989-9455. They also have an excellent Web site: www.choices.org. Another good Web site with information for other countries is www.growthhouse.org. (A note for those of you living outside the United States: The information in this chapter deals with specific legal documents that may differ in your country. However, the issues discussed are universal. As you read, take what is useful to you and skip over the rest.) Let us start with some definitions.

A durable power of attorney is a document that *appoints another person to act in your place if you are unable to do so.* It differs from a living will in two ways. A living will is good only in case of a terminal illness, while a durable power of attorney for health care can apply to any illness. Second, a durable power of attorney for health care allows you to appoint another person to act for you. A living will does not allow for this provision. For example, when parents go on trips they often leave a friend or other family member with the power of attorney so that someone can take care of any emergency that might happen with the children. A durable power of attorney for *health care* is a document in which you appoint someone else to act as your agent concerning health care. In other words, it allows someone else to make decisions for you. It does not give the person the right to act in other ways such as handling your financial matters. This document is activated only when for some reason you are unable to make decisions yourself (e.g., when in a coma or mentally incompetent).

Besides naming someone as your agent, the durable power of attorney can give *guidelines* to your agent about your *wishes concerning health care*. You do not have to give guidance to your agent. However, many people wish to do so. This guidance indicates almost anything you want done for your care; it may range from use of aggressive life-sustaining measures to the withholding of life-sustaining measures.

To complete a durable power of attorney for health care means making many decisions.

First, you must decide who will be your agent. This can be a friend or member of the family. It cannot be the physician who is providing your care. There are some considerations to be made in choosing your agent. This person should generally be available in the geographic area where you live. If the agent is not available to make decisions for you, he or she is not much help. Just to be on the safe side, you can also name a back-up agent who would act in your behalf if your primary agent was not available. Second, you must be sure that this person thinks like you think or at least would be willing to carry out your wishes. Third, the person must be someone who you feel would be able to carry out your wishes. Sometimes a spouse or child is not the best agent because this person is too close to you emotionally. For example, if you wished not to be resuscitated in the case of a severe heart attack, your agent has to be able to tell the doctor not to resuscitate. This could be very difficult or impossible for a family member to decide then and there. Be sure the person you choose as your agent is up to this task and would not say "do everything you can" at this critical time. Finally, you want your agent to be someone who will not find this job too much of an emotional burden. Thus, the person has to be comfortable with the role, as well as willing and able to carry out your wishes.

In review, look for these characteristics in an agent:

- Someone who is likely to be available should they need to act on your behalf.
- Someone who understands your wishes and is willing to carry them out.
- Someone who is emotionally prepared and able to carry out your wishes.
- Someone who will not be emotionally burdened by carrying out your wishes.

169

As you can see, finding the right agent is a very important task. This may mean talking to several people. These may be the most important interviews that you ever conduct. We will talk more about discussing your wishes with family, friends, and your doctor later.

The other major decision you may want to make is what you want to put in your durable power of attorney for health care. In other words, what are your directions to your agent? Some forms give several general statements of desires concerning medical treatment.

For example:

> *I do not want my life to be prolonged and I do not want life-sustaining treatment to be provided or continued: (1) if I am in an irreversible coma or persistent vegetative state; or (2) if I am terminally ill and the application of life-sustaining procedures would serve only to artificially delay the moment of my death; or (3) under any other circumstances where the burdens of the treatment outweigh the expected benefits. I want my agent to consider the relief of suffering and the quality as well as the extent of the possible extension of my life in making decisions concerning life-sustaining treatment.*

> *I want my life to be prolonged and I want life-sustaining treatment to be provided* unless I am in a coma or vegetative state *which my doctor reasonably believes to be irreversible. Once my doctor has reasonably concluded that I will remain unconscious for the rest of my life, I do not want life-sustaining treatment to be provided or continued.*

I want my life to be prolonged to the greatest extent possible without regard to my condition, the chances I have for recovery or the cost of the procedures.

If you use a form containing such suggested general statements, all you need to do is to initial the statement that best applies to you.

Other forms make a *"general statement of granted authority,"* in which you give your agent the power to make decisions. However, you do not write out the details of what these decisions should be. In this case, you are trusting your agent to follow your wishes. Since these wishes are not explicitly written, it is very important that you have discussed them in detail with your agent.

All forms also have a space in which you can write out any specific wishes. You are not required to give specific details but may wish to do so.

Knowing what details to write is a little complicated because none of us knows the exact circumstances in which the agent will have to act. However, you can get some idea by asking your doctor about what he thinks might be the most likely things to happen to someone with your condition. Then you can direct your agent on how to act. Your specific directions can discuss outcomes, specific circumstances, or both. If you discuss outcomes, then the statement should focus on what types of outcomes would be acceptable and which would not. For example, "resuscitate if I can continue to fully function mentally." The following are some of the more common specific circumstances that are encountered with major chronic diseases.

- Alzheimer's disease and other neurologic problems are diseases that can leave you with little or no mental function. As we said earlier, these are generally not life-threatening, at least not for many years. However, things happen to these patients that can be life-threatening, such as pneumonia and heart attacks. What you need to do is decide how much treatment you want. For example, do you want antibiotics if you get pneumonia? Do you want to be resuscitated if your heart stops? Do you wish a feeding tube if you are unable to feed yourself? Remember, it is your choice as to how you answer each of these questions. You may not want to be resuscitated but may want a feeding tube. If you want aggressive treatment, you may want to use all means to sustain life, or, more conservatively, you may not want any special means used to sustain life. For example, you may want to be fed but may not want to be placed on life-support equipment.

- You have a very bad lung function that will not improve. Should you be unable to breathe on your own, do you want to be placed in an intensive care unit on mechanical ventilation (a breathing machine)? Remember, in this case you will not improve. To say that you never want ventilation is very different from saying that you don't want it if it is used to sustain life when no improvement is likely. Obviously, mechanical ventilation can be life-saving in cases such as a severe asthma attack when it is used for a short time until the body can regain its normal function. Here, the issue is not whether to use mechanical ventilation ever but, rather, when or under what circumstances you wish it to be used.

- You have a heart condition that cannot be improved with angioplasty (cleaning out the arteries) or surgery. You are in the cardiac intensive care unit. If your heart stops functioning, do you want to be resuscitated? Like artificial ventilation, the question is not "Do you ever want to be resuscitated?" but, rather, "Under what conditions do you or do you not want resuscitation?"

171

From these examples it is hoped that you can begin to identify some of the directions that you might want to give in your advance directive or durable power of attorney for health care. Again, to understand these better or to make them more personal to your own condition, you might want to talk with your physician about what the common problems and decisions are for people like you.

In summary, there are several decisions you need to make in directing your agent on how to act in your behalf.

- Generally, *how much treatment do you want?* This can range from the very aggressive, that is, doing many things to sustain life, to the very conservative, which is doing almost nothing to sustain life, except to keep you clean and comfortable.
- Given the types of life-threatening things that are likely to happen to people with your condition, *what sorts of treatment do you want and under what conditions?*
- If you become *mentally incapacitated*, what sorts of treatment do you want for *other illnesses* such as pneumonia?

Many people get this far. That is, they have thought through their wishes about dying and have even written them down in a durable power of attorney for health care. This is an excellent beginning but not the end of the job. A good manager has to do more than just write a memo. He or she has to see that the memo gets delivered. If you really want your wishes carried out, it is important that you share them fully with your agent, your family, and your doctor. This is often not an easy task. In the following section, we will discuss ways to make these conversations easier.

Before you can have a conversation, all interested parties need to have copies of your durable power of attorney for health care. Once you have completed the documents, have them witnessed and signed. You can have your Durable Power of Attorney notarized instead of having it witnessed. Make several copies at any copy center. You will need copies for your agent(s), family members, and your doctor. It does not hurt also to give one to your lawyer.

Now you are ready to talk about your wishes. Nobody likes to discuss their own death or that of a loved one. Therefore, it is not surprising that when you bring up this subject the response is often "Oh, don't think about that," or "That's a long time off," or "Don't be so morbid, you're not that sick." Unfortunately, this is usually enough to end the conversation. Your job as a good self-manager is to keep the conversation open. There are several ways to do this. First, plan on how you are going to begin your discussion of this subject. Here are some suggestions.

Prepare your durable power of attorney, and then *give copies* to the appropriate family members or friends. *Ask them to read it* and then set a specific time to *discuss it*. If they give you one of those responses we talked about earlier, say that you understand this is a difficult topic, but that it is important to you that you discuss it with them. This is a good time to practice the "I" messages discussed in Chapter 10. For example, "I understand that death is a difficult thing to talk about. However, it is very important to me that we have this discussion."

You might get *blank copies* of the durable power of attorney forms for all your family members and suggest that *you all fill them out and share them*. This could even be part of a family get-together. Present this as an important aspect of being a mature adult and family member. Making this a family project in which everyone is involved may make it easier to discuss. Besides, it will help to clarify everyone's values about the topics of death and dying.

If these two suggestions seem too difficult, or, for some reason, are impossible to carry out, you might *write a letter* or prepare an *audiotape* that can then be sent to members of your family. In the letter or tape, talk about why you feel your death is an important topic to discuss and that you want them to know your wishes. Then state your wishes, providing reasons for the choices you indicate. At the same time, send them a copy of your durable power of attorney for health care. Ask that they respond in some way or that you set aside some time to talk in person or on the phone with them.

Of course, in deciding on your agent, it is important that you choose someone with whom you can talk freely and exchange ideas. If your chosen agent is not willing to or is unable to talk to you about your wishes, then you have probably chosen the wrong agent. Also, don't be fooled. Just because someone is very close does not mean that he or she really understands your wishes or would be able to carry them out. This is not a topic that should be left to a mutual, unspoken understanding unless you don't mind if they decide differently from what you wish. For this reason, choosing someone who is not as close to you emotionally is sometimes better. Talking with your agent is especially important if you have not written details of your wishes.

Talking with Your Doctor

From our research, we have learned that, in general, people have a much more difficult time talking to their doctors about their wishes surrounding death than to their families. In fact, only a very small percentage of people who have written durable powers of attorney for health care, or other advance directives, ever share these with their physician.

There are several reasons why it is important that this discussion take place. First, *you need to be sure that your doctor has values that are compatible with your wishes.* If you and your doctor do not have the same values, it may be difficult for him or her to carry out your wishes. Second, *your doctor needs to know what you want.* This allows him or her to take appropriate actions such as writing orders to resuscitate or not to use mechanical resuscitation should this be needed. Third, *your doctor needs to know who your agent is and how to contact this person.* If an important decision has to be made and your wishes are to be followed, the doctor must talk with your agent.

It is important to give your doctor a copy of your durable power of attorney for health care, so that it can become a permanent part of your medical record. Again, the problem is often how to start this conversation with the doctor.

As surprising as it may seem, many physicians also find this a very difficult topic to discuss with their patients. After all, they are in the business of helping to keep people alive and well. They don't like to think about their patients dying. On the other hand, most doctors want their patients to have durable powers of attorney for health care. This relieves them of pressure and worry.

If you wish, *plan a time with your doctor when you can discuss your wishes.* This should not be a side conversation at the end of a regular visit. Rather, start a visit by saying, "I want a few minutes to discuss with you my wishes in the event of a serious problem or impending death." When put in this way, most doctors will make time to talk with you. If the doctor says that he or she does not have enough time, then ask when you can make another appointment to talk with him or her. This is a situation in which you may need to be a little assertive. Sometimes a doctor, like your family members or friends, might say, "Oh, you don't have to worry about that, let me do it," or "We'll worry about that when the time comes." Again, you will have to take the initiative, using an "I" message to communicate that this is important to you and you do not want to put off the discussion.

Sometimes doctors do not want to worry you. They think they are doing you a favor by not describing all the unpleasant things that might happen to you or the potential treatments in case of serious problems. You can help your doctor by telling him or her that having control and making some decisions about your future will ease your mind. Not knowing or not being clear on what will happen is more worrisome than being faced with the facts, unpleasant as they may be, and dealing with them.

Even knowing all of the above, it is still sometimes hard to talk with your doctor. Therefore, it might also be helpful to *bring your agent* with you when you have this discussion. The agent can facilitate the discussion and, at the same time, meet your doctor. This also gives everyone a chance to clarify any misunderstandings about your wishes. It opens the lines of communication so that if your agent and physician have to act to carry out your wishes they can do so with few problems. If somehow you just "can't" talk with your doctor, at least mail him or her a copy of your durable power of attorney. This way it will become part of your medical records.

So now you have done all the important things. You can rest easy. The hard work is over. However, remember that you can change your mind at any time. Your agent may no longer be available, or your wishes might change. Be sure to keep your durable power of attorney for health care updated. Like any legal document, it can be revoked or changed at any time. In all cases, it *must be updated every seven years.* However, if you are incapacitated when your durable power of attorney for health care expires, it will remain in effect until you can renew it. The decisions you make today are not forever.

Please note: Many states recognize durable powers of attorney for health care that are created in another state. However, this is not always the case. As of now, this is an unclear legal issue. To be on the safe side, if you move or spend a lot of time in another state, it is best to check with a lawyer in that state to see if your document is legally binding there.

Be sure to check on the appropriate forms for your state by asking your doctor or lawyer or by writing to Choice In Dying.

174

Community Resource Detective's Kit

Durable Power of Attorney for Health Care

Choice In Dying

Senior Center

Hospital, Health Care Organization

Growth House

Making your wishes known about how you want to be treated in case of serious or life-threatening illness is one of the most important tasks of self-management. The best way to do this is to prepare a durable power of attorney for health care and share this with your family, close friends, and physician.

A few more notes about preparing for death:

In most parts of the United States, as well as in many other parts of the world, hospice care is available. In everyone's life there comes a time when medical care is no longer helpful and we need to prepare for death. Today, we often have several weeks or months to make these preparations. This is when hospice care is so very useful. The aim of hospice care is to provide the terminally ill patient with the highest quality of life possible. At the same time, hospice professionals help both the patient and the family prepare for death with dignity and also help the surviving family members. Today most hospices are "in home" programs. This means that the patient stays in his or her own home and the services come to them. In some places there are also residential hospices where people can go for their last days.

One of the problems with hospice care is that often people wait until the last few days before death to ask for this care. They somehow see asking for hospice as "giving up." By refusing hospice care, they often put an unnecessary burden on themselves, friends, and family.

Hospice care can be most useful for the months before death. Most hospices only accept people who are expected to die within six months. This does not mean that you will be thrown out if you "outlive" your time. Six months is a guideline, not a fixed time. The message here is that if you, a family member, or a friend is in the ending stage of illness, find and utilize your local hospice. It is a wonderful final gift.

• • •

Suggested Further Reading

Cantor, Norman L. *Advance Directives and the Pursuit of Death With Dignity*. Bloomington: Indiana University Press, 1993.

King, Nancy M. P. *Making Sense of Advance Directives*. Washington, D.C.: Georgetown University Press, 1996.

176

CHAPTER
13

Healthy Eating

177

D EVELOPING HEALTHY EATING HABITS IS IMPORTANT FOR EVERYONE. We
know that a nutritionally balanced eating plan not only gives us more
energy and endurance to be able to carry out our activities, but also
makes us feel good and reduces our risk for certain health problems.
While food alone cannot prevent or cure a chronic disease, learning to
make healthier choices in the foods we eat can help us manage symptoms, prevent complications, and feel more in control of our health.

Changing our eating habits, however, is not easy. What we eat and how we
prepare it are habits that have developed over years. For many of us, they are an
important part of our family and cultural traditions. Therefore, suddenly trying to
change everything about the way we eat is not only unrealistic, but unnecessary
and unpleasant as well. If we want to make healthful changes in our eating habits
that will last over time, and perhaps become the new practices we pass on to others, then these changes need to be small and gradual.

In this chapter, we offer some suggestions on how to begin making changes in
our eating habits and how to enjoy doing it. We have included tips for planning
well-balanced meals, making healthier food choices, managing a healthy weight,
and minimizing some of the problems commonly associated with eating and
weight management. Just like any of the other self-management techniques discussed in this book, healthy eating will help you take control of your health.

What Is Healthy Eating?

Healthy eating does not mean that you can never eat your favorite foods again
or that you have to "diet" or buy "special" foods. Rather, it means learning to
make healthier choices in the foods you eat, finding new or different ways to prepare these foods, and eating in moderation.

You can start eating healthier by following these basic principles: eating a variety of foods, eating regular meals, and trying to eat the same amount of food at each meal.

Eating a variety of foods is important so the body gets all the essential nutrients it needs to function well. These nutrients include protein, carbohydrates, fats, vitamins, and minerals. Each plays an important role and can be found in varying amounts in the different food groups. Taking vitamins and food supplements can never replace eating a variety of foods. These "extras" contain only the nutrients we know about. To get all essential nutrients (both known and unknown), we need to eat a variety of foods.

Eating regularly and eating breakfast every day provides the body with the fuel it needs to function well throughout the day. For this reason, it is best to space your meals and/or snacks out during the day, remembering to include breakfast. Breakfast is important because it is the first source of energy for the body after a long night of fasting. Deciding how to space the meals will depend on an individual's needs. Some people may do well with three regular meals spaced four to five hours apart, while others who cannot eat as much at a meal may need to eat smaller, more frequent meals or snacks during the day.

Eating the same amount at each meal also ensures that the body has an adequate supply of energy to function optimally throughout the day. Not eating enough at a meal or skipping meals can throw your system off and lead to habits such as snacking on sweets or "junk" food. It can also aggravate symptoms or cause other problems, such as irritability or mood swings and low blood sugar, or *hypoglycemia*. Eating too much can cause problems as well, such as indigestion or increased discomfort or pain from difficulties in breathing when the stomach becomes distended and the diaphragm is crowded. Eating too much at the evening meal can also contribute to weight gain and poor sleep.

Planning a Healthy Meal

By now, most of us know that an eating plan that is low in fat and high in fiber is healthy for everyone. But many of us have difficulty putting this into practice when planning and preparing meals. Therefore, we have provided the following simple formula and sample food guide to help you plan and prepare healthier meals and snacks.

A Formula for Healthy Meals

This general formula for a healthy meal not only offers variety, but also encourages us to eat more servings of vegetables and fruit (at least five a day), as well as to choose more appropriate portion sizes for the foods we include in our regular meals.

PROTEINS are made from amino acids that are used by the body after being broken down when digested. Proteins are the building blocks for the enzymes and hormones that help regulate bodily functions. They are needed to maintain the body's immune system, which helps fight infection and build or repair damaged tissues. Proteins also provide energy for the body. Our bodies produce some proteins, but not all the ones it needs to carry out all functions. Therefore, we must get these proteins from the foods we eat. Meat, fish, poultry, eggs, and dairy products provide us with complete proteins. Vegetable sources of protein such as legumes, grains, nuts, and seeds are incomplete proteins; however, when eaten in the right combinations, vegetable sources can form complete proteins. Vegetable proteins provide additional health benefits because they are lower in fat and high in fiber and contain no cholesterol.

CARBOHYDRATES are the major source of energy for the body's muscles and metabolism. For this reason they should make up the majority of the foods and calories we eat each day. There are a variety of different foods that contain carbohydrates. These include starches, or *complex carbohydrates,* such as grains, rice, pasta, breads, legumes (peas and beans), root plants (potatoes, carrots, etc.), and other vegetables. Grains and vegetables also provide an excellent source of fiber. There are also *simple carbohydrates,* or sugars, which are found in fruits and some dairy products. These too are good sources of carbohydrate. Less desirable sources of carbohydrates include processed products or foods that are made with refined or table sugar, honey, syrups, and jellies; these sources provide calories but have little or no nutritional value.

FATS consist of substances called fatty acids and glycerol, which binds the fatty acids together. They can be saturated, monounsaturated, or polyunsaturated. Fats are used by the body for energy. While our bodies need some fat to help build, strengthen, and repair tissues, excess fat from the foods we eat is stored by the body, leading to weight gain and increased risk of heart disease. Meat, whole-milk dairy products, nuts, seeds, peanuts, and oils are rich sources of fat. Because fats contain twice the number of calories per gram than do proteins or carbohydrates, it is recommended we limit the amount of fat we eat, especially the saturated fats that come from animal sources or that are found in processed foods. Limiting foods that are high in saturated fat also helps to reduce dietary cholesterol, which is not a fat but tends to be present in high-fat dairy products, meats, and poultry.

VITAMINS AND MINERALS are necessary in small amounts to help build strong bones and muscles and to ensure that the body functions properly. They are found in varying amounts in the different foods we eat. Therefore, if we eat a variety of foods, chances are we are getting the vitamins and minerals we need. Depending on our health needs, however, some people may need to take supplements, not to take the place of a balanced eating plan, but to help us reach the recommended daily allowance of certain vitamins and/or minerals. If supplements are needed, select one that contains 50–100% of the recommended daily allowance (or recommended nutrient intake) for the various vitamins and minerals. Examples include Centrum, One-a-Day, Unicap, as well as the generic store brands. There is no need to take higher doses or "megadoses" of supplements unless prescribed and supervised by the doctor. Too much of some vitamins or minerals can create health problems and even some toxic reactions.

A healthy or well-balanced meal should include

- **One portion of protein (21–35 grams/serving):** Examples of proteins from the accompanying food guide include meat, poultry, fish, milk products, grains, and legumes or tofu. Meat portions should be about the size of the palm of your hand and ½ to 1 inch (1 to 2 cm) thick. Consider those choices that are lower in fat.

- **One or more portions of vegetables that are low in starch or carbohydrates (5 grams/serving):** Portion sizes on these vegetables are not limited, and they can be eaten as often as you like. Examples from the guide include leafy green vegetables, tomatoes, broccoli, cucumber, etc.

- **Two portions of grain products and/or vegetables that are high in starch or carbohydrates (15 grams/serving):** These foods include breads, rice, pasta, legumes, corn, potatoes, carrots, etc. Portion sizes may need to be limited for these foods if you are counting carbohydrates and/or calories. (For portion sizes, see the accompanying food guide.)

- **One portion of fruit (which is higher in carbohydrates—15 grams/serving):** Portion sizes for fruit are also limited if you are counting carbohydrates and/or calories.

- **Moderate use or avoidance of foods that are high in fat, sugar, and sodium**, such as dressings, sweets, salty snacks, alcohol, soft drinks, relishes, jams, and jellies.

Reading Food Labels

Reading and understanding food labels can also help us make healthier food choices. The majority of the foods we buy have labels that list the nutritional content of those products. These are called *Nutrition Facts,* and there are usually many different ones listed on the package. A few of the most important ones to consider are the serving or portion size, number of servings per package, total carbohydrates, total fat, cholesterol, and sodium. The example on page 187 outlines more specifically what to look for. On some packages of food products, the label may be too small to list the nutritional content; however, the manufacturer still needs to provide this information. Therefore, there is usually a telephone number or address on the label you can call or write to for this information.

FOOD GUIDE

Formula for Healthy Eating

One portion of PROTEINS + one portion of VEGETABLES + one portion of FRUIT
+ two portions of STARCH/CARBOHYDRATES

PROTEINS: One portion exchange = proteins, fats, and carbohydrates

	Portion		Portion
CHEESE: *(0 g carbohydrates, 7 g protein per oz; grams fat varies)*		**MEATS:** *(0 g carbohydrates, 7 g protein per oz)*	
Fresh (Mexican) cheese	**2–3 oz**	Lean 0–3 g fat per oz: round, sirloin, flank, steak, tenderloin	**2–3 oz**
Cottage cheese (low fat)	**¼ cup**	Medium-fat 5 g fat per oz: ground beef, corned beef, prime rib	**2–3 oz**
Regular cheese (8 g fat per oz)	**2–3 oz**	High-fat 8 g fat per oz: sparerib, ground pork, pork sausage	**2–3 oz**
MILK: *(12 g carbohydrates, 8 g protein; grams fat varies)*		**POULTRY: chicken, turkey, hen** *(0 g carbohydrates, 7 g protein per oz)*	
Milk, nonfat, low fat	**1 cup**	Lean 0–3 g fat : white meat, skinless breast	**2–3 oz**
Powdered milk	**3 tbsp.**	Medium-fat 5 g fat: dark meat, leg or thigh with skin	**2–3 oz**
Whole milk	**1 cup**	High-fat 8 g fat: fried chicken with skin, duck	**2–3 oz**
Soy milk	**1 cup**		
YOGURT: *(20 g carbohydrates, 8 g protein)*		**PROCESSED MEAT/LUNCH MEAT:**	
Yogurt (low fat, varies)	**1 cup**	Low-fat: turkey, ham, beef, hot dogs, hamburger meat *(high in sodium)*	**2–3 oz**
EGGS: *(0 g carbohydrates, 7 g protein)*			
Fresh eggs *(high in cholesterol)*	**1 egg**	**ORGAN MEATS:** *(high in cholesterol)*	
		Liver, tripe, brains, tongue, etc.	**2–3 oz**
NOTE:			
Meat portions: Measured by the size of the palm of your hand and ½ to 1 inch (1 to 2 cm) thickness		**OTHER:**	
		Tofu *(0 g carbohydrates, 7 g protein, 3 g fat)*	**½ cup**
FISH: *(0 g carbohydrates, 7 g protein per oz)*		Peanut butter *(0 g carbohydrates, 7 g protein, 8 g fat)*	**2 tbsp.**
Lean 0–3 g fat per oz: Cod, halibut, flounder, haddock, trout, tuna, salmon, sardines, oysters on the half shell, shrimp	**2–3 oz**		
Medium-fat 5 g fat per oz: Any fried fish	**2–3 oz**		

(continues)

FOOD GUIDE
Formula for Healthy Eating (continued)

VEGETABLES LOW IN STARCH:
One portion exchange = 5 g carbohydrate, 2 g protein

Portion*		Portion

Vegetables low in starch can be eaten as often as you like

Fresh, Frozen or Canned (low sodium)*

Artichoke	Green onion or scallions	
Asparagus	Nopales (Cactus)	
Broccoli	Mushrooms	
Brussel sprouts	Okra	
Bean sprouts	Onions	
Cabbage, Chinese cabbage	Peppers (red and green)	
Celery	Radish	
Chayote (vegetable pear)	Salad greens	
Chicory	Squash	
Chilies, spicy	Spinach	
Cucumber	Tomato	
Cauliflower	Turnips	
Eggplant (aubergine)	Watercress	
Garlic	Zucchini	
Green beans		

Vegetable Juices

Mixed vegetables (V-8)	½ cup
Tomato	¼ cup

FREE FOOD LIST:
(Contains less than 5 g of carbohydrates per serving)

DRINKS

Atol (cornmeal drink)	1 cup
Bouillon or broth (chicken or beef)	
Bouillion or broth, low sodium	1 cup
Carbonated or mineral water	
Club soda	
Cocoa powder (3 tsp.)	1 cup

DRINKS (continued)

Coffee	
Diet soft drinks, sugar-free	1 cup
Drink mixes, sugar-free	
Horchata (rice drink)	½ cup
Tea	
Tonic water, sugar-free	

* Foods listed without a serving size can be eaten as often as you like

FOOD GUIDE
Formula for Healthy Eating (continued)

STARCHY VEGETABLES:
One portion exchange = 15 g carbohydrate, 3–7 g protein, 0–1 g fat (if oil added)

	Portion		Portion
Beans, lentils, peas	½ cup	Snow peas	½ cup
Beets	½ cup	Squash, winter	½ cup
Carrots	½ cup	*Yam, sweet potato	½ cup
Corn	½ cup	*Yautia	½ cup
Jicama	½ cup		
Plantain	½ cup	* 1 small or ½ cup	
*Potato, baked or boiled	1 cup		

STARCH/CARBOHYDRATES:
One portion exchange = 15 g carbohydrate, 3 g protein, 0–1 g fat

PASTA, CEREALS AND GRAINS

		BREAD	
Bran cereals	½ cup	Roll, regular	½
Cereals, unsweetened	¾ cup	White, whole wheat	1 slice
Granola, low fat	¼ cup	Bread (made of milk/salt, small)	½
Oats, plain	½ cup	English muffin, plain	½
Rice Krispies	½ cup	Hot dog or hamburger bun	½
Wheat germ	3 tbsp.	Pancake, regular, low fat	1
Pasta	½ cup	Pita bread, 6 inches across	½
Rice, cooked	½ cup	Tortilla, corn, regular	1
		Tortilla, flour, medium	1
		Waffle, regular, low fat	1

FATS:
One portion exchange = 5 g fat

MONOUNSATURATED FAT

Avocado, medium	¼	Peanut butter, crunchy	2 tbsp.
Nuts:		Olives, all types (large)	5
almonds, cashews	6 nuts	Sesame seeds	1 tsp.
peanuts	8 nuts		
pecans, walnuts	4 halves		

(continues)

FOOD GUIDE
Formula for Healthy Eating (continued)

FRUITS:
One portion exchange = 15 g carbohydrate

Fresh	Portion		Portion
Apple, small	1	Peach, medium	1
Apricots, medium	2	Plum, small	1
Banana, small	½	Tangerine, medium	1
Berries: strawberries, blueberries	1 cup	Watermelon	½ cup
Coconut, fresh (shredded)	½ cup	**Canned Fruit**	
Dates	3	Low fat/ Low sugar	½ cup
Figs, large	2	Regular	¼ cup
Grapefruit, small	½ cup	**Dried Fruit**	
Grapes, small	½ cup	Figs, apricots	2
Guava, medium	2	Raisins	2 tbsp.
Kiwi, large	1	**Fruit Juices (sugar free, or low in sugar)**	
Lemon, large	1	Apple	½ cup
Lime, large	1	Apricot nectare	½ cup
Mango, small	1	Carbonated juice drinks	½ cup
Melon, honeydew	¼	Fruit punch	½ cup
Orange, small	1	Grapefruit	½ cup
Papaya, small	¼	Orange	½ cup
Pineapple	½ cup	Sweet juices (low sugar)	½ cup
Pear, small	1	Tamarindo	½ cup
Persimmons, medium	1		

PROBLEM FOODS:
Some fats can raise blood cholesterol levels and artificial sugars raise glucose levels

POLYUNSATURATED FATS		SATURATED FATS	
Margarine, low fat	1 tsp.	Bacon	1 slice
Mayonnaise, regular	1 tsp.	Butter, regular	1 tsp.
Mayonnaise, reduced fat	1 tsp.	Butter, reduced fat	1 tbsp.
Miracle Whip	1 tbsp.	Coconut, sweetened (shredded)	2 tbsp.
Oil (corn, safflower, soybean)	1 tsp.	Cream, half and half	2 tbsp.
Salad dressing	1 tbsp.	Sour cream, regular	2 tbsp.
Seeds (pumpkin, sunflower)	1 tsp.	Sour cream, reduced fat	3 tbsp.
		Shortening or lard	2 tbsp.

184

FOOD GUIDE
Formula for Healthy Eating (continued)

PROBLEM FOODS:
Some fats can raise blood cholesterol levels and sugars raise glucose levels

	Portion		Portion
DESSERTS/SWEETS		Syrup (sugar-free)	**2 tbsp.**
Cake with frosting	**1 slice**	Tamal, small	**1**
Danish, small	**1**		
Flan, with milk	**½ cup**	**ALCOHOLIC BEVERAGES**	
Fruit tart or pie	**1 slice**	Beer	**12 oz**
Honey	**1 tbsp.**	Champagne	**4 oz**
Jam or jelly (low sugar or light)	**2 tbsp.**	Liquor	**1 oz**
Rice pudding	**½ cup**	Wine	**4 oz.**

FREE FOOD LIST:
Contains less than 5 g of carbohydrates per serving

SUGAR-FREE FOODS		Gum (sugar-free)
Candy, hard (sugar-free)	**1 candy**	Sugar substitutes
Gelatin dessert (sugar-free)		
Gelatin, unflavored		

Recommendations:

+ Recommended portion of sodium is 400 mg

* Foods listed without a serving size can be eaten as often as you like

• Sugar substitutes, alternatives, or replacements that are approved by the Food and Drug Administration (FDA) are safe to use. Common brand names include:

Equal® (aspartame)	Sprinkle Sweet® (saccharin)
Sweet One® (acesulfame K)	Sweet-10® (saccharin)
Sugar Twin® (saccharin)	Sweet 'n Low® (saccharin)

Abbreviations for the measurement units:

Grams	g	Tablespoon	tbsp.
Teaspoon	tsp.	Ounce	oz
Milligrams	mg		

Eating Tips for People with Specific Chronic Conditions

Please note that this formula for healthy eating is a general guideline that is applicable to almost everyone; however, each individual may have slightly different needs, depending on age, gender, body size, activity level, health, likes and dislikes, and even the availability or affordability of certain foods. The following are some specific recommendations for people with different chronic diseases.

Diabetes

For people with diabetes, it is important to limit the amount of carbohydrates that you eat. The carbohydrates are what break down into glucose. This glucose, with the help of insulin, passes into the cells to provide energy for the body. However, in diabetes, this process does not work well and can cause complications. Therefore, if you have diabetes it is necessary to reduce or limit the amount of foods you eat that contain carbohydrates. The recommended amount of carbohydrates for each regular meal is between 45 and 60 grams. These can come from varied sources that are listed in the food guide on pages 181–185. The amount of carbohydrates (in grams) per suggested portion or serving size is also provided. This should help you to count carbohydrates for each meal.

In addition, because people with diabetes have an increased risk of developing heart disease, circulatory problems, and hypertension, it is also important to reduce the amount of fat, cholesterol, and sodium in the foods you eat. Reducing fat can also help with weight loss and, therefore, help lower your blood sugar. (See the tips for reducing fat and increasing fiber in the boxes on page 188.) Even a small weight loss of 5–10 pounds (2–4 kg) can make a big difference in your blood sugar level.

Heart Disease

For people with heart disease, it is very important to reduce the amount of fat and cholesterol in the foods you eat and to increase your fiber intake. This helps to prevent the narrowing and hardening of the arteries that can cause heart attacks. Reducing fat also helps to control your blood pressure and weight. In the same way, reducing your salt and sodium intake helps to prevent or control high blood pressure (hypertension). The food guide also lists some of the problem foods that are higher in fat, cholesterol, and sodium to help you make healthier choices. The tips mentioned on page 188 also provide suggestions for ways to reduce fat and increase fiber in your eating plan.

Lung Disease

For people with lung disease, especially emphysema, it is sometimes necessary to increase the amount of protein you eat. This helps increase your energy,

Nutrition Facts to Look for on Food Labels

- The **serving size** and **servings per container** are important. Many products have more than one serving or portion per package. Also, it is possible that even the amount in one serving is more than what is recommended for certain nutrients. (This example is 1 serving size, and there is 1 serving per container.)

- The amount of **total carbohydrates** is listed **per serving**, not package, which is 39 g in this example. This includes the amount of **fiber** (2 g) as well as **sugars** (2 g) in or added to the product. This fact is especially important for individuals watching or counting their carbohydrates.

- The amount of **total fat** (7 g in this example) includes saturated fat (3.5 g) and unsaturated fat (not listed). For individuals watching their fat intake, the total fat should be 5 grams per serving. Look for products with less saturated fat.

- Be aware of the amount of **cholesterol** (15 mg in this example). Lower is better. Products with less saturated fat also have less cholesterol.

- Note the amount of **sodium** (890 mg in this example). The recommended amount is less than 400 mg per serving.

Nutrition Facts

Serving Size 1 Entree (227 g)
Serving Per Container 1

Amount Per Serving

Calories 250   Calories from Fat 60

	% Daily Value*
Total Fat 7 g	11%
Saturated Fat 3.5 g	17%
Cholesterol 15 mg	5%
Sodium 890 mg	37%
Total Carbohydrate 39 g	13%
Dietary Fiber 2 g	8%
Sugars 2 g	
Protein 8 g	

Vitamin A 20%	Vitamin C 15%
Calcium 10%	Iron 6%

*Percent Daily Values are based on a 2,000 calorie diet.

Tips for Reducing Fat in Your Eating Plan

- Eat more poultry and fish, less red meat with a moderate size portion (2–3 oz, or 50–100 g, which is about the size of a deck of cards or the palm of your hand).
- Choose leaner cuts of meat.
- Trim off the outside fat and remove the skin from poultry.
- Eat egg yolks and organ meats (liver, kidneys, brains) in moderation.
- Broil, barbecue, or roast meats instead of frying them.
- Avoid deep-fried foods.
- Skim fat off stews and soups.
- Use low-fat or nonfat milk and milk products.
- Use added fats such as butter, margarine, oils, gravy, sauces, and salad dressings sparingly in food preparation (no more than 3–4 teaspoons [15–20 mL] per day).
- Use a nonstick pan with cooking oil spray.

Tips for Increasing Fiber in Your Eating Plan

- Build your meals around vegetables, grain products, and fruits.
- Eat a variety of fruits and vegetables, raw or slightly cooked.
- Eat low-fat grain products such as whole-wheat breads, brown or whole-grain rice, and corn tortillas.
- Eat more beans and rice or lentils as meat substitutes.
- Snack on fruit or nonfat yogurt, not sweets, pastries, or ice cream.
- Drink plenty of water to help move the fiber through your system.

strength, and resistance. Also, people who have difficulty eating enough to maintain an adequate amount of nutrients may need to eat foods that contain more protein and calories than normally recommended. The food guide lists several different sources of protein. Also, the section "Common Problems with Gaining Weight" (page 198) lists some suggestions for increasing the amount of nutrients and calories in your eating plan.

If you have specific concerns about your eating plan, consult with your doctor or a nutritionist to help you choose which tips are appropriate for you, or adjust some of these recommendations to meet your unique health needs.

189

Managing a Healthy Weight[1]

Achieving and/or maintaining a healthy weight is important for everyone. Weight can have a considerable impact on your disease symptoms and your ability to exercise or otherwise manage health problems. Therefore, finding a healthy weight and maintaining it are important parts of the self-management process. But what is a healthy weight?

A healthy weight is *not* an "ideal" weight. There is no such thing as an "ideal" weight for an individual. The tables of "ideal" weights are only general guidelines for weight ranges based on population statistics. These tables should *not* be used to define your specific weight. Being at a healthy weight does *not* mean being "skinny" like the popular images portrayed in the media. These body shapes and weights are not realistic for most of us. In fact, being too thin sometimes contributes to health problems.

A healthy weight is one whereby you reduce your risk of developing health problems, or further complicating existing ones, *and* feel better both mentally and physically. Finding a healthy weight depends on several factors, such as your age, your activity level, how much of your weight is fat, where the fat is on your body, and whether or not you have weight-related medical problems such as high blood pressure or a family history of such problems. You may already be at a healthy weight and need only to maintain it by eating well and staying active. Consult your doctor to help you determine what a healthy weight is for you, given your condition and treatment needs.

The decision to change weight is a very personal one. To help you decide whether or not you are ready to make any changes, ask yourself the following questions:

---

[1] Portions of this chapter have been adapted from two publications: *Thinking About Losing Weight?* Northern California Regional Health Education Center, Kaiser Permanente Medical Care Program, 1990. *The Weight Kit.* Stanford Center for Research in Disease Prevention, Health Promotion Resource Center, Stanford University, 1990.

Why Change My Weight?

The reasons for losing or gaining weight are different for each individual. The most obvious reason may be your physical health, but there may also be psychological or emotional reasons for wanting to change. Examine for yourself why you want to change.

For example, changing my weight will help me . . .

- ❏ Lessen my disease symptoms (e.g., pain, fatigue, shortness of breath) and control blood sugar
- ❏ Give me more energy to do the things I want to do
- ❏ Feel better about myself
- ❏ Change the way others perceive me
- ❏ Feel more in control of my disease and/or my life

If you have other reasons, jot them down here:

_____

_____

_____

What Will I Have to Change?

Two ingredients for successful weight management are developing an active lifestyle and making changes in your eating patterns. Let's look closely at what each of these involves.

An active lifestyle implies doing some physical activity that burns calories and regulates appetite and metabolism, both important for weight management. Physical activity can also help you develop more strength and stamina, as well as move and breathe more easily. In other words, activity doesn't wear you down or out, but actually boosts your energy level. You will find much more information about exercise and tips for choosing activities that suit *your* needs and lifestyle in Chapters 6 through 9.

Making changes in your eating habits starts by making small, gradual changes in what you eat. This may mean changing the emphasis on or quantity of certain foods you eat. You will find tips for doing this at the beginning of the chapter.

While most of us are concerned with losing weight and keeping it off, some people with chronic disease struggle to gain or maintain a healthy weight. If you experience a continual or extreme weight loss because your disease or treatment interferes with your appetite and/or depletes your body of valuable nutrients (such as protein, vitamins, and minerals), you may need to work at gaining weight.

Some common problems associated with making changes in your eating habits and/or weight management are discussed on pages 192–201.

You can also find more information on healthy eating in the references listed at the end of this chapter. Particularly useful is the USDA's *Eating Right the Dietary Guidelines Way.*

Am I Ready to Change for Good?

Success is important in weight management. Therefore, the next step is to evaluate whether or not you are ready to make these changes. If you are not ready, you may be setting yourself up for failure and those nasty weight "ups and downs." This is not only discouraging but unhealthy as well. For this reason it is helpful to plan ahead by considering the following types of questions:

- Is there someone or something that will make it easier for you to change?

- Are there problems or obstacles that will keep you from becoming more active or changing the way you eat?

- Will worries or concerns about family, friends, work, or other commitments affect your ability to carry out your plans successfully at this time?

Looking ahead at these factors can help you find ways to build support for desired changes, as well as minimize possible problems you may encounter along the way. Use the accompanying chart to help you identify some of these factors.

After you have examined these things, you may find that now is not the right time to start anything. If it is *not, set a date in the future* for a time when you will reevaluate these changes again. In the meantime, accept that this is the right decision for you at this time, and focus your attention on other goals.

If you decide that now *is* the right time, start by changing those things that feel *most comfortable to you.* You don't have to do it all right away. Remember, slow and steady wins the race.

To help get started, keep track of what you are currently doing. For example, write down your daily routine to identify where you might be able to add some exercise. Or keep a food diary for a week to see what, when, why, and how much you eat. This can help you identify how and where to make changes in your eating habits, as well as how to shop for and prepare meals. The diary may also help you look at the relationship between your eating patterns and emotions or other symptoms. The sample food–mood diary on page 193 may be useful. Next, choose only one or two things to change first. Allow yourself time to get used to these and then add more changes. The goal setting and action planning skills discussed in Chapter 2 will help with this.

191

Things That Will Enable Me to Make the Desired Changes	Things That Will Make it Difficult for Me to Change
Example: I have the support of family and friends.	*Example:* The holidays are coming up and there are too many gatherings to prepare for.

192

Common Problems with Eating for Health

"I enjoy eating out (or I hate to cook), so how do I know if I'm eating well?"

Whether it's because you don't have time, you hate to cook, or you just don't have the energy to go grocery shopping and prepare meals, eating out may suit your needs. This is not necessarily bad if you know which choices are healthy ones.

Here are tips on eating out:

- Select restaurants that offer variety and flexibility in types of food and methods of preparation. Feel free to ask what is in a dish and how it is prepared, especially if you are eating in a restaurant where the dishes are new or different from what you are used to.

Food–Mood Diary

Date	Time	What I Ate	Where I Ate	Mood/Feelings

- Plan what type of food you will eat and how much. (You can bring the leftovers home.)

- Choose items low in fat, sodium, and sugar or ask if they can be prepared that way. For example, appetizers might include steamed seafood or raw vegetables without fancy sauces or dips, or bread without butter. You may request salad with dressing on the side, or bring your own oil-free dressing. For an entree, you might try broiled, barbecued, baked, grilled, or steamed dishes. Choose fish or poultry over red meat. Avoid breaded, fried, sauteed, or creamy dishes. Choose dishes whose ingredients are listed. Instead of a whole dinner, consider ordering a la carte and lots of vegetables (without butter or sauces). For dessert, select fruit, nonfat yogurt, or sherbet. You might split an entree or a dessert with someone else.

- Order first so that you aren't tempted to change your order after hearing what others have selected.

- If you want fast food, choose salads with dressing on the side, baked potatoes instead of fries, juice or milk instead of soda, and frozen yogurt instead of ice cream.

"I snack while I watch TV (or read)."

If you know this is a problem for you, plan ahead by preparing healthier snacks. For example, rather than eating "junk" food like chips and cookies, munch on fresh fruit, raw vegetables, or air-popped popcorn. Try designating specific areas at home and work as "eating areas" and limit your eating to those areas.

"I eat when I'm bored/depressed/feeling lonely, etc."

Many people find comfort in food. Some people eat when they don't have any-thing else to do or just to fill in time. Some eat when they're feeling down or both-ered. Unfortunately, at these times, you often lose track of what and how much you eat. These are also the times when celery sticks, apples, or popcorn never seem to do the trick. Instead, you start out with a full bag of potato chips and, by the end of an hour, have only crumbs left. To help control these urges, try to

- Keep a food-mood diary. Every day, list what, how much, and when you eat. Note how you are feeling when you have the urge to eat. Try to spot patterns so you can anticipate when you will want to eat without really being hungry. (The sample diary on page 193 can be used for this.)

- Make a plan for when these situations arise. If you catch yourself feeling bored, go for a short walk, work on a jigsaw puzzle, or otherwise occupy your mind and hands. This may be a time to practice a distraction technique.

"Healthy food doesn't taste the same as real food. When I eat, I want something with substance, like meat and potatoes! The healthy stuff just doesn't fill me up!"

Just because you are trying to make healthier food choices does not mean that you will never again eat meat and potatoes. It only means that you will change some of the ways you prepare these foods, as well as what you buy at the store. Some of these tips were already discussed on page 188. Additional information is available in the references at the end of this chapter.

195

"But I LOVE to cook!"

If you love to cook, you are in luck. This is your opportunity to take a new cooking class or to buy a new recipe book on healthy cooking. Again, experiment with different ways to modify your favorite recipes, making them lower in fat, sugar, and sodium.

"I'm living alone now, and I'm not used to cooking for one. I find myself over-eating so food isn't wasted."

This can be a problem, especially if you are not used to measuring ingredients. You may be overeating or eating a "second dinner" to fill time. Or maybe you are one of those people who will eat for as long as the food is in front of you. Whatever the reason, here are some ways to help you to deal with the extra food:

- Don't put the serving dishes on the table. Take as much as you feel you can comfortably eat and bring only your plate to the table.

- As soon as you've finished eating, wrap up what you haven't eaten and put it in the refrigerator or freezer. This way, you have leftovers for the next day or whenever you don't want to cook.

- Invite friends over for dinner once in a while so that you can share food and each other's company, or plan a potluck supper with neighbors or relatives.

- Join a community kitchen or attend a community or church supper.

Common Problems with Losing Weight

"Gosh, I wish I could lose ten pounds in the next two weeks. I want to look good for . . . ."

Sound familiar? Most everyone who has tried to lose weight wants to lose it quickly. This is a hard pattern to break because, although it may be possible to lose 5 to 10 pounds (2–5 kg) in one or two weeks, it is not healthy nor is it likely to stay off. Rapid weight loss is usually water loss, which can be dangerous, causing the body to become dehydrated. When this happens you may also experience other symptoms such as light-headedness, headaches, fatigue, and poor sleep. Rather than doing this to yourself, try a different approach—one employing realistic goal setting and positive self-talk. (These are discussed in greater detail in Chapters 2 and 5, respectively.) Here are some approaches to sensible weight loss:

- Set your goal to lose weight *gradually,* just one or two pounds (1 kg) a week.

- Identify the specific steps you will take to lose this weight, for example, increasing activities and/or changing what you eat.

- Change your self-talk from "I really need to lose 10 pounds right away" to "Losing this weight gradually will help me keep it off for good."

- Be patient. You didn't gain weight overnight, so you can't expect to lose it overnight.

"I can lose the first several pounds relatively painlessly, but I just can't seem to lose those last few pounds."

This can be frustrating and puzzling, especially when you have been eating healthy and staying active. However, it is quite common and usually means that your body has adapted to your new calorie intake and activity level. While your first impulse may be to cut your calorie intake even further, it probably won't help and could be unhealthy. Remember, you want to make changes you can live with.

Ask yourself how much of a difference one, two, or even five pounds will really make. If you are feeling good, chances are you don't need to lose more weight. It is not unhealthy to live with a few extra pounds, if you are staying active and eating low-fat foods. You may already be at a healthy weight given your body size and shape. Also, you may be replacing fat with muscle, which weighs more. However, if you decide that these pounds must go, try the following:

196

- Modify your goal so that you maintain your weight for a few weeks; try to lose a pound more gradually over the next few weeks.

- Try adding to your physical activity exercise goals, especially if the current activity you do has become easy. Increasing your activity level will help you to use more calories and maintain your muscle mass. Less weight will be stored in the form of fat. (Tips for safely increasing your exercise are found in Chapter 6.)

- Again, be patient and allow your body time to adjust to your new patterns.

197

"I always feel so deprived of the foods I love when I try to lose weight."

The key to reaching and maintaining a healthy weight is to make changes you can tolerate, even enjoy. This means they must suit your lifestyle and needs. Unfortunately, when thinking about losing weight, most of us tend to think of all the things we *can't* eat. Change this way of thinking now! There are probably as many (if not more) enjoyable foods you CAN eat than ones you should limit. Sometimes it is just a matter of learning to prepare foods differently, rather than eliminating them completely. If you like to cook, this is your opportunity to become creative, learning new recipes or finding ways to change old ones. There are many good cookbooks on the market today to help you make this process more enjoyable. Some of these tips were outlined on page 188 of this chapter, and more can be found in the references listed at the end of the chapter.

"I eat too fast or I finish eating before everyone and find myself reaching for seconds."

Eating too fast happens for a couple of reasons. One may be that you are limiting yourself to only two or three meals a day, not eating or drinking between meals. This can leave you so hungry at mealtime that you practically inhale your food. Another reason may be that you have not had a chance to slow down and relax before eating. Slowing down your eating can help you decrease the amount of food you eat. If you find you are too hungry, feeling stressed out, or in a hurry, try one or more of the following:

- Try not to skip meals. In this way you are less likely to overeat at the next meal.

- Allow yourself to snack on healthy foods between meals. In fact, plan your snacks for mid-morning and afternoon. Keep a banana, some raw vegetables, or a few crackers with you for those "snack attacks."

- Eat more frequent, smaller meals. This may also be easier on your digestive system, which won't be overwhelmed by a large meal eaten in a hurry.

- Chew your food well. Food is an enjoyable necessity! Chewing your food well also eases the burden on your digestive system.

- Drink plenty of water! Six to eight glasses of water per day is recommended. This helps you to eat less and helps prevent medication side effects, aids elimination, and keeps the kidneys functioning properly.

- Try a relaxation method about a half hour before you eat. Several methods are discussed in Chapter 5.

198

Common Problems with Gaining Weight

"I don't know how to add pounds."

Here are some ways to increase the amount of calories and/or nutrients you eat. Unfortunately, these may also add some fat to your eating plan. Check with your doctor or a nutritionist to see which of the following tips are appropriate for you.

- Eat smaller meals more often during the day.
- Don't skip meals.
- Eat high-calorie foods first at each meal, saving the vegetables, fruits, and beverages for later.
- Snack on calorie-rich foods such as avocados, nuts, seeds, nut butter, or dried fruits.
- Drink high-calorie beverages such as shakes, malts, fruit whips, and eggnogs.
- Eat high-protein foods from lean-protein sources (see the food guide on pages 181–185 for ideas).
- Use milk to prepare creamed dishes with meat, fish, or poultry.
- Add meat to salads, soups, and casseroles.
- Add milk or milk powder to sauces, gravies, cereals, soups, and casseroles.
- Use melted cheese on vegetables and other dishes.

- Add butter, margarine, oils, and creams to dishes (1–3 table-spoons [15–45 mL] per day).

- Use protein, vitamin, and mineral supplements if needed (consult with your doctor or a nutritionist).

"Food doesn't taste as good as before."

If you have had a tracheostomy, are receiving oxygen through a nasal cannula, or are taking certain medications, you may have noticed a decrease in your taste sensations. To compensate, you may have also noticed that you've been increasing the amount of salt you add to your foods. Be careful of this because a high sodium intake can cause water retention or "bloating," which can result in increased blood pressure. To avoid this, try enhancing the flavors of foods by

- Experimenting with herbs, spices, and other seasonings. Start with just about ¼ teaspoon (5 mL) in a dish for four people.

- Modifying recipes to include a wide variety of ingredients to make the food look and taste more appealing.

- Chewing your food well. This will allow the food to remain in your mouth longer and provide more stimulation to your taste buds.

If the decline in taste is keeping you from getting essential nutrients, you may need to adjust the calorie content of these foods. Tips for doing this are mentioned above.

"It takes so long to prepare meals. By the time I'm done, I'm too tired to eat."

If this is a problem for you, then it's time to develop a plan, because you need to eat to maintain your energy level. Here are some hints to help:

- Plan your meals for the week.

- Then go to the grocery store and buy everything you will need.

- Break your food preparation into steps, resting in between.

- Cook enough for two, three, or even more servings, especially if it's something you really like.

- Freeze the extra portions in single-serving sizes. On the days when you are really tired, thaw and reheat one of these pre-cooked, frozen meals.

- Ask for help, especially for those big meals or at family gatherings.

"Sometimes eating causes discomfort." Or, "I'm afraid I'll become short of breath while I'm eating."

People who experience shortness of breath or who find it difficult and physically uncomfortable to eat meals tend to eat less and may be underweight. For some, eating a large meal causes indigestion. Indigestion, along with a full stomach, reduces the space your breathing muscles have to expand and contract. This can aggravate breathing problems. If this is a problem for you:

200

- Try eating four to six smaller meals a day, rather than the usual three larger meals. This reduces the amount of oxygen you need to chew and digest each meal.

- Avoid foods that produce gas or make you feel bloated. You can determine which foods affect you this way by trying different foods and observing the results. Often these foods include vegetables such as cabbage, broccoli, brussels sprouts, varieties of onions, beans, and fruits like raw apples, melons, and avocados, especially if eaten in large quantities.

- Eat slowly, taking small bites and chewing your food well. You should also pause occasionally during a meal. Eating quickly to avoid an episode of shortness of breath can actually bring one on. Slowing down and breathing evenly reduces the amount of air you swallow while eating.

- Practice a relaxation exercise about half an hour before mealtime, or take time out for a few deep breaths during the meal.

"I can't eat much in one sitting."

There is no real need to eat only three meals a day. In fact, for many it is recommended that you eat four to six smaller meals. If you choose to do this, include "no fuss," high-calorie snacks like milk, bread, and fruits or liquid protein shakes as part of these extra meals. If you still can't finish a whole meal, be sure to eat the portion of your meal that is highest in calories first. Save the vegetables, fruits, and beverages for last.

Common Problems with Maintaining Your Weight

"I've been on a LOT of diets before and lost a lot of weight. But I've always gained it back, and then some. It's so frustrating, and I just don't understand WHY this happens!!!"

Many of you have probably experienced this problem, which occurs because the diet was short-term and calorie-restricted; it did not emphasize changes in eating habits. In fact, this is the problem with many "diets." They involve such drastic changes in both what is eaten and the way it is eaten that they cannot be tolerated for long. Because your body does not know when more food will be available again, it reacts physiologically to this deprivation, slowing its metabolism to adapt to a smaller amount of food energy. Then, when you've had enough of the diet, or have lost the weight and return to your old eating habits, you gain the weight back. Sometimes you even gain back more weight than you lost. Again, the body is responding physiologically, replenishing its stores, usually in the form of fat. This fat serves as a concentrated energy source to be called upon again when calories are restricted. This causes the weight to go up and down in cycles which, as mentioned before, is unhealthy and very discouraging.

This situation is further complicated by feelings of deprivation, as you probably had to give up your favorite foods. Therefore, when you reach your goal weight, you begin to eat all of those foods again freely and most likely in larger quantities.

The key to maintaining a healthy weight is developing healthy eating habits that are enjoyable to you and fit into your lifestyle. We have already discussed many of these tips earlier in this chapter. Here are a few more:

- Set a small weight-range goal that you consider to be healthy for *you*. Weights fluctuate naturally. By setting a range, you will allow yourself some flexibility.

- Monitor your activity level. Once you have lost some weight, exercise three to five times a week to improve your chances of keeping the weight off. If possible, gradually increase your activity level.

"I do okay maintaining my weight for a short time. Then something happens beyond my control, and my concerns about what I eat become insignificant. Before I know it I've slipped back into my old eating habits."

If you had only a little slip, don't worry about it. Just continue as if nothing happened. If the slip is longer, try to evaluate why: Is there a situation or circumstance requiring a lot of attention now? If so, weight management may be taking a back seat for a while. This is okay. The sooner you realize this the better, and try to set a date when you will start your weight management program again. You may even want to join a support group and stay with it for at least four to six months. If so, look for one that

- Emphasizes good nutrition and the use of a wide variety of foods.

- Emphasizes changes in eating habits and patterns.
- Gives support in the form of ongoing meetings or long-term follow-up.

Eating well does not mean that you are forever forbidden to eat certain foods. It means learning to eat a variety of foods in the right quantities to maintain your health and/or better manage your disease symptoms. This involves changing your eating patterns and emphasizing foods that are *lower* in fat, sugar, and sodium. These changes are also important for effective weight management. If you choose to make some of the changes suggested in this chapter, remember that you should not feel like you are punishing yourself, nor that this is a life sentence to boring, bland food. As a self-manager, it's up to you to find the changes that are best for you. And if you experience setbacks, identify the problems and work at resolving them. Remember, if you *really* want to, you *can* do it!

• • •

Community Resource Detective's Kit

Nutrition Information

U.S. Department of Agriculture, Room 325-A, 6505 Belcrest Rd., Hyattsville, MD 20782

Public Library

Local Health Library

Public Health Department

Agricultural Extension Service

Local Heart Association

Local Dietetic Association

Local Cancer Society

Local Diabetes Association

Local Health Center or Clinic

Suggested Further Reading

General

American Heart Association. *An Active Partnership for the Health of Your Heart.* Dallas: American Heart Association, 1990.

Brody, Jane. *Jane Brody's Nutrition Book.* New York: Bantam, 1982.

Deutsch, Ronald M., and Judi S. Morrill, Ph. D. *Realities of Nutrition.* Rev. ed. Palo Alto, Calif.: Bull Publishing, 1993.

Escott-Stump, Sylvia. *Nutrition and Diagnosis-Related Care.* Philadelphia, Pa.: Lea and Febiger, 1988.

Peters, James A., Kenneth Burke, and Debra White. "Nutrition and the pulmonary patient." In *Pulmonary Rehabilitation: Guidelines to Success*, edited by John E. Hodgkin, Eileen G. Zorn, and Gerilynn L. Conners. Stoneham, Mass.: Butterworth Publishers, 1984.

Williams, Sue R. S. *Essentials of Nutrition and Diet Therapy.* St. Louis, Mo.: Times Mirror/Mosby College Publishing, 1990.

United States Department of Agriculture. *Eating Right the Dietary Guidelines Way.* Hyattsville, Md.: U.S. Department of Agriculture, Human Nutrition Information Service, 1990.

Vegetarian Eating

Lappé, Frances. *Diet for a Small Planet.* New York: Ballantine, 1985.

Robertson, Laurel, Carol Flinders, and Bronwen Godfrey. *Laurel's Kitchen: A Handbook for Vegetarian Cookery and Nutrition.* New York: Bantam, 1978.

Weight Control

Breitrose, P. *The Weight Kit.* Stanford Center for Research in Disease Prevention, The Health Promotion Resource Center, Stanford University, 1990.

Ferguson, James M. *Habits Not Diets.* 2nd ed. Palo Alto, Calif.: Bull Publishing, 1988.

Nash, Joyce D. *Maximize Your Body Potential.* Palo Alto, Calif.: Bull Publishing, 1986.

Nelson, Miriam E. *Strong Women Stay Slim.* New York: Bantam Books, 1998.

Waltz, Julie. *Food Habit Management: A Comprehensive Guide to Dietary Change.* Edmonds, Wash.: Northwest Learning Associates, 1982.

Managing Your Medicines

H AVING A CHRONIC ILLNESS USUALLY MEANS TAKING ONE OR MORE MEDICA-
TIONS. Thus a very important management task is to understand your
medications and to use them appropriately. This chapter will help you do
just that.

A Few General Words About Medications

Almost nothing receives as much advertising as medications. If we read a magazine, listen to the radio, or watch TV, we see a constant stream of ads, all aimed
to convince us that if we just use this pill or potion our symptoms will be cured.
"Recommended by 90% of the doctors asked." "Take an aspirin for your
headache." Almost as a backlash to this advertising, we have been taught to avoid
excess medications. We have all heard about or experienced some of the ill effects
of medications. "Just say no to drugs." "Drugs can kill." It is all very confusing.

Your body is its own healer and, if given time to work, most common symptoms and disorders will improve. The prescriptions filled by the body's internal
pharmacy are frequently the safest and most effective treatment. So patience, careful self-observation, and monitoring are excellent therapeutic choices.

It is also true that medications can be a very important part of managing a
chronic illness. These medications do not cure the disease. They generally have
one or more of the following purposes.

1. *They relieve symptoms through their chemical actions.* For example, an inhaler delivers medications that help expand the
   bronchial tubes and make it easier to breathe, or a nitroglycerin
   tablet expands the blood vessels allowing more blood to reach
   the heart, quieting angina.

2. Other medications are aimed at *preventing further problems.* For example, medications that thin the blood help prevent blood clots, which cause strokes and heart problems.

3. A third type of medication *helps to improve the disease or slow the disease process.* For example, nonsteroidal anti-inflammatory drugs can help arthritis by quieting the inflammatory process. Likewise, digitalis can help regulate and strengthen the heart beat.

206

4. Finally, there are medications to *replace substances that the body is no longer producing adequately.* This is how insulin is used by someone who is diabetic.

In all cases, the purpose of medication is to lessen the consequences of disease or to slow its course. You may not be aware that the medications are doing anything. For example, if a drug is slowing the course of the disease, you may not feel anything, and this may lead you to believe that the drug isn't doing anything. It is important to continue taking your medications, even if you cannot see how they are helping. If this concerns you, ask your doctor.

We pay a price for having such powerful tools. Besides being helpful, all medications have undesirable side effects. Some are predictable and minor, and some are unexpected and life-threatening. From 5% to 10% of all hospital admissions are due to drug reactions.

What Is a Side Effect?

A side effect is *any* effect other than the one you want. Usually, it is an undesirable effect. Some side effects are stomach problems, constipation or diarrhea, sleepiness or dizziness. It is important to know the common side effects for the medications you take. Sometimes people say they can't or won't take a drug because of possible side effects. This is a reasonable response. However, before making a decision to stop taking a drug or refusing to take it, there are some questions you should ask yourself and your doctor.

Are the benefits from this medication more important than the side effects?

The use of chemotherapy for people with cancer is a good example. While these drugs have side effects, many people still choose the drugs because of their life-saving qualities. To take or not to take a drug is your decision. However, it should always be looked upon as "will I be better off with the drug despite its side effects?"

Are there some ways of avoiding the side effects or making them less severe?

Many times the way you take the drug, for example, with food or without food, can make a difference. Ask your doctor or pharmacist for advice on this question.

Are there other medications with the same benefits but fewer side effects?

Often there are several drugs that do the same thing but react differently in different people. Unfortunately, no one knows how a drug will react in you until you have taken it. Therefore, your doctor may have to try several medications before hitting on the one that is best for you. For this reason, when getting a new medication, it is always best to ask for a prescription for only a week or two with a refill for a month. In this way, if the drug does not work out, you will not have had to pay for what you do not use.

Taking Multiple Medications

It is not uncommon for patients with multiple problems to be taking multiple medications: a medication to lower blood pressure, anti-inflammatory drugs for arthritis, a pill for angina, a bronchodilator for asthma, antacids for heartburn, a tranquilizer for anxiety, plus a handful of over-the-counter remedies and herbs. *Remember, the more medications you are taking, the greater the risk of adverse reactions.* Fortunately, it is often possible to reduce the number of medications and the associated risks. It requires forging an effective partnership with your doctor. This involves participation in determining the need for the medication, selecting the medication, properly using the medication, and reporting back to your doctor the effect of the medication.

An individual's response to a particular medication varies depending on age, metabolism, activity level, and the waxing and waning of symptoms characteristic of most chronic diseases. Many medications are prescribed on an as-needed ("PRN") basis so that you need to know when to begin and end treatment and how much medication to take. You need to work out a plan with your doctor to suit your individual needs.

For most medications, *your doctor depends on you* to report what effect, if any, the drug has on your symptoms and what side effects you may be experiencing. Based on that critical information your medications may be continued, increased, discontinued, or otherwise changed. In a good doctor–patient partnership, there is a continuing flow of information. There are important things you need to let your doctor know and critical information you need to receive.

Unfortunately, this vital interchange is too often shortchanged. Studies indicate that fewer than 5% of patients receiving new prescriptions asked any questions of their physicians or pharmacists. Doctors tend to interpret patient silence as understanding and satisfaction with the information received. Mishaps often occur because patients do not receive adequate information about medications and don't understand how to take them or fail to follow instructions given to them. Safe, effective drug use depends on your understanding of the proper use, the risks, and the necessary precautions associated with each medication you take. *You must ask questions.*

208

Many patients are reluctant to ask their doctor questions, fearing to appear ignorant or to be challenging the doctor's authority. But asking questions is a necessary part of a healthy doctor–patient relationship.

The goal of treatment is to maximize the benefit and minimize the risks. This means taking the fewest medications, in the lowest effective doses, for the shortest period of time. Whether the medications you take are helpful or harmful often depends on how much you know about your medications and how well you communicate with your doctor.

What You Need to TELL Your Doctor

Even if your doctor doesn't ask, there is certain vital information you should mention to her or him.

Are you taking any medications?

Report to your physician and dentist *all* the prescription and nonprescription medications you are taking, including birth control pills, vitamins, aspirin, antacids, laxatives, and herbal remedies. This is especially important if you are seeing more than one physician. Each one may not know what the others have prescribed. Knowing all the medications and herbs you are taking is essential to correct diagnosis and treatment. For example, if you have symptoms like nausea or diarrhea, sleeplessness or drowsiness, dizziness or memory loss, impotence or fatigue, they may be due to a drug side effect rather than a disease. It is critical for your doctor to know what medications you are taking to help avoid problems from drug interactions. It is helpful to carry an up-to-date list with you or at least know the names and dosages of all the medications you are taking. Saying that you are taking "the little green pills" usually doesn't help identify the medication. Sometimes it is beneficial to bring in all your medications (including over-the-counter medications) in a bag so that your doctor can review them, advising you which to continue and which to stop or discard. You can also write a list of all the medications you are taking and their dosages. In this way your doctor doesn't have to spend valuable minutes looking through your medical chart.

Have you had allergic or unusual reactions to any medications?

Describe any symptoms or unusual reactions you have had to any medications taken in the past. Be specific: which medication and exactly what type of reaction. A rash, fever, or wheezing that develops after taking a medication is often a true allergic reaction. If any of these develop, call your doctor at once. Nausea, ringing in the ears, light-headedness, agitation, and so on, are likely to be side effects rather than true drug allergies.

Do you have any major chronic diseases or other medical conditions?

Many diseases can interfere with the action of a drug or increase the risk of using certain medications. Diseases involving the kidneys or liver are especially important to mention since these diseases can slow the metabolism of many drugs and increase toxic effects. Your doctor may also avoid certain medications if you now or in the past have had such diseases as hypertension, peptic ulcer disease, asthma, heart disease, diabetes, or prostate problems. Also be sure to let your doctor know if you are possibly pregnant or are breast-feeding since many drugs cannot be safely used in those situations.

What medications were tried in the past to treat your disease?

If you have a chronic disease, it is a good idea to keep your own written record of what medications were tried in the past to manage the condition and what the effects were. Knowing your past responses to various medications will help guide the doctor's recommendation of any new medications. However, just because a medication did not work successfully in the past does not necessarily mean that it can't be tried again. Diseases change and may become more responsive to treatment.

What You Need to ASK Your Doctor

Do I really need this medication?

Some physicians decide to prescribe medications not because they are really necessary, but because they think patients want and expect drugs. Physicians often feel pressure to do something for the patient, so they reach for the prescription pad. Don't pressure your physician for medications. If your doctor doesn't prescribe a medication, consider that good news rather than a sign of rejection or disinterest. Ask about herbs and other nondrug alternatives. Many conditions can be treated in a variety of ways, and your physician can explain alternative choices. In some cases lifestyle changes such as exercise, diet and stress management should be considered before making a choice. When any treatment is recommended, also ask what the likely consequences are if you postpone treatment. Sometimes the best medicine is none at all.

210

What is the name of the medication?

If a medication is prescribed, it is important that you know its name. Write down both the brand name and the generic (or chemical) name. If the medication you get from the pharmacy doesn't have the same name as the one your doctor prescribed, ask the pharmacist to explain the difference.

What is the medication supposed to do?

Your doctor should tell you why the medication is being prescribed and how it might be expected to help you. Is the medication intended to prolong your life, completely or partially relieve your symptoms, or improve your ability to function? For example, if you are given a diuretic for high blood pressure, the medication is given primarily to prevent later complications (i.e., stroke or heart disease) rather than to stop your headache. On the other hand, if you are given an aspirin, the purpose is to help ease the headache. You should also know how soon you should expect results from the medication. Drugs which treat infections or inflammation may take several days to a week to show improvement, while antidepressant medications and some arthritis drugs typically take several weeks to begin working.

How and when do I take the medication and for how long?

Understanding how much of the medication to take and how often to take it is critical to the safe, effective use of medications. Does "every six hours" mean "every six hours while awake"? Should the medication be taken before meals, with meals, or between meals? What should you do if you accidentally miss a dose? Should you skip it, take a double dose next time, or take it as soon as you remember? Should you continue taking the medication until the symptoms subside or until the medication is finished?

The answers to such questions are very important. For example, if you are taking a nonsteroidal anti-inflammatory drug for arthritis, you may feel better within a few days, but should still take the medication as prescribed to maintain the anti-inflammatory effect. Or, if you abruptly stop taking steroid medications used for severe asthma as soon as the wheezing improves, you are likely to relapse. If you are using an inhaled medication for treatment of asthma, the way you use the inhaler critically determines how much of the medication actually gets into your lungs. Taking the medication properly is vital. Yet when patients are surveyed, nearly 40% report that they were not told by their physicians how to take the medication or how much to take. If you are not sure about your prescription, call your doctor. Such calls are never considered a bother.

What foods, drinks, other medications, or activities should I avoid while taking this medication?

The presence of food in the stomach may help protect the stomach from some medications while it may render other drugs ineffective. For example, milk products or antacids block the absorption of the antibiotic tetracycline, so this drug is best taken on an empty stomach. Some medications may make you more sensitive to the sun, putting you at increased risk for sunburn. Ask whether the medication prescribed will interfere with driving safely. Other drugs you may be taking, even over-the-counter drugs and alcohol, can either amplify or inhibit the effects of the prescribed medication. Taking aspirin along with an anticoagulant medication can result in enhanced blood-thinning and possible bleeding. The more medications you are taking, the greater the chance of an undesirable drug interaction. So ask about possible drug-drug and drug-food interactions.

What are the most common side effects, and what should I do if they occur?

All medications have side effects. You need to know what symptoms to be on the lookout for and what action to take if they develop. Should you seek immediate medical care, discontinue the medication, or call your doctor? While the doctor cannot be expected to tell you every possible adverse reaction, the more common and important ones should be discussed. Unfortunately, a recent survey showed that 70% of patients starting a new medication did not recall being told by their physicians or pharmacists about precautions and possible side effects. So it may be up to you to ask.

Are there any tests necessary to monitor the use of this medication?

Most medications are monitored by the improvement or worsening of symptoms. However, some medications can disrupt body chemistry before any telltale symptoms develop. Sometimes these adverse reactions can be detected by laboratory tests such as blood counts or liver function tests. In addition, the levels of some medications in the blood need to be measured periodically to make sure you are getting the right amounts. Ask your doctor if the medication being prescribed has any of these special requirements.

212

Can an alternative or generic medication that is less expensive be prescribed?

Every drug has at least two names, a generic name and a brand name. The generic name is the name used to refer to the medication in the scientific literature. The brand name is the company's unique name for the drug. When a drug company develops a new drug in the United States, it is granted exclusive rights to produce that drug for 17 years. After this 17-year period has expired, other companies may market chemical equivalents of that drug. These generic medications are generally considered as safe and effective as the original brand-name drug, but often cost half as much. In some cases, your physician may have a good reason for preferring a particular brand. Even so, if cost is a concern, ask your doctor if there is a less expensive, but equally effective, medication available. Sometimes you can save money by purchasing your medications through the mail. Many Health Maintenance Organizations and the American Association of Retired Persons offer mail-order prescription services. We are also beginning to see medication sales through the Internet. It pays to check around for the best prices.

Is there any written information about the medication?

Realistically, your doctor may not have time to answer all of your questions in great detail. Even if your physician carefully answers the questions, it is difficult for anyone to remember all of this information.

Fortunately, there are many other valuable sources of information you can turn to: pharmacists, nurses, package inserts, pamphlets, and books. Several particularly useful books to consult are listed at the end of this chapter.

A Special Word About Pharmacists

Pharmacists are an underutilized resource. They have gone to school for many years to learn about medications, how they act in your body, and how they interact with each other. Your pharmacist is an expert on medications. You can often call him or her on the phone. In addition, many hospitals, medical schools, and schools of pharmacy have medication information services where you can call and ask your questions. As a self-manager, don't forget pharmacists. They are important and helpful consultants.

Remembering to Take Your Medicine

No matter what medication is prescribed, it won't do you any good if you don't take it. Nearly half of all medicines are not taken regularly as prescribed. There are many reasons why this occurs: forgetfulness, lack of clear instructions, complicated dosing schedules, bothersome side effects, cost of the medications, and so on. Whatever the reason, if you are having trouble taking your medications as prescribed, discuss this with your doctor. Often, simple adjustments can make it easier. For example, if you are taking five different medications, sometimes one or more can be eliminated. If you are taking one medication three times a day and another four times a day, your doctor may be able to simplify the regimen, perhaps even prescribing medications that you need to take only once or twice a day. Understanding more about your medications, including how they can help you, may also help motivate you to take them regularly.

If forgetting to take your medications is a major problem, then here are some suggestions:

- *Place the medication or a reminder* next to your toothbrush, on the meal table, in your lunch box, or in some other place where you're likely to "stumble over" it. (But be careful where you put the medication if children are around.) Or you might put a reminder note on the bathroom mirror, the refrigerator door, the coffee maker, the television, or some other conspicuous place. If you link taking the medication with some well-established habit like meal times or watching your favorite television program, you'll be more likely to remember.

- *Make a medication chart* containing each medication you are taking and when you take it; or check off each medication on a calendar as you take it. You might also *buy a "medication organizer"* at the drugstore. This container separates pills according to the time of day they should be taken. You can fill the organizer once a week so that all of your pills are ready to take at the proper time. A quick glance at the organizer lets you know if you have missed any doses and prevents double dosing.

- *Get a watch that can be set to beep at pill-taking time.* There are also "high-tech" medication containers available that beep at a pre-programmed time to remind you to take your medication.

- *Ask other family or household members to help remind you* to take your medications.

- *Don't let yourself run out* of your medicines. When you get a new prescription, mark on your calendar the date a week before your medications will run out. This will serve as a reminder to get your next refill. Don't wait until the last pill.

If you plan to travel, *put a note on your luggage reminding you* to pack your pills. Also, *take along an extra prescription* in your carry-on luggage in case you lose your pills or your luggage.

Self-Medication

In addition to medications prescribed by your doctor, you, like most people, may take nonprescription or over-the-counter (OTC) medications and herbs. In fact, within every two-week period nearly 70% of people will self-medicate with one or more drugs. Many OTC drugs are highly effective and may even be recommended by your doctor. But if you self-medicate, you should know what you are taking, why you are taking it, how it works, and how to use medications wisely.

More than 200,000 nonprescription drug products are offered for sale to the American public, representing about 500 active ingredients. An estimated $8 billion is spent on such products. Nearly 75% of the public receives its education on OTC drugs solely from TV, radio, newspaper, and magazine advertising. Unfortunately, many of the claims for drugs are either not true or subtly misleading.

You need to be aware of the barrage of drug advertising aimed at you. The implicit message of such advertising is that for every symptom, every ache and pain, every problem, there is a product solution. While many of the OTC products are effective, many are simply a waste of your money and a diversion of your attention from better ways of managing your illness.

If you self-medicate, here are some suggestions:

- *Always read drug labels and follow directions carefully.* The label must by law include names and quantities of the active ingredients, precautions, and adequate directions for safe use. Careful reading of the label, including review of the individual ingredients, may help prevent you from ingesting medications that have caused problems for you in the past. If you don't understand the information on the label, ask a pharmacist or doctor before buying it.

- *Do not exceed the recommended dosage or length of treatment* unless discussed with your doctor.

- *Use caution if you are taking other medications.* Over-the-counter and prescription drugs can interact, either canceling or exaggerating the effects of the medications. If you have questions about drug interactions, ask your doctor or pharmacist before mixing medicines.

- Try to *select medications with single active ingredients* rather than the combination ("all-in-one") products. In using a product with multiple ingredients, you are likely to be getting drugs for symptoms you don't even have, so why risk the side effects of medications you don't need? Single-ingredient products also allow you to adjust the dosage of each medication separately for optimal symptom relief with minimal side effects.

- When choosing medications, *learn the ingredient names* and try to *buy generic products.* Generics contain the same active ingredient as the brand-name product, usually at a lower cost.

- *Never take or give a drug from an unlabeled container* or a container whose label you cannot read. Keep your medications in their original labeled containers or transfer them to a labeled medication organizer or pill dispenser. Do not make the mistake of mixing different medications in the same bottle.

- *Do not take medications left over* from a previous illness or that were prescribed for someone else, even if you have similar symptoms. Always check out medications with your doctor.

- Pills can sometimes get stuck in the esophagus, the "feeding tube." To help prevent this, be sure to *drink at least a half glass of liquid* with your pills and remain standing or sitting upright for a few minutes after swallowing.

- If you are pregnant or nursing, have a chronic disease, or are already taking multiple medications, *consult your doctor* before self-medicating.

- *Store your medications in a safe place* away from the reach of any children. Poisoning with medications is a common and preventable problem. The bathroom medicine chest is not automatically a particularly secure or dry place to store medications. Consider a lockable tool chest or fishing box.

- Many medications have an expiration date of about two to three years. *Dispose of all expired medications.*

Medications can help or harm. What often makes the difference is the care you exercise and the partnership you develop with your doctor.

• • •

Suggested Further Reading

Consumer Reports Books. *The Complete Drug Reference.* Yonkers, N.Y.: Consumers Union.

Holmes, H. Nancy. *Taking Your Medications Safely.* Springhouse Publishing Co., 1996.

Rybacki, Janet J., and James W. Long. *The Essential Guide to Prescription Drugs.* New York: HarperCollins, 1999.

Silverman, Harold. *The Pill Book,* 8th ed. New York: Bantam Doubleday, 1998.

CHAPTER 15

Understanding Chronic Lung Disease

SHORTNESS OF BREATH, TIGHTNESS IN THE CHEST, WHEEZING, PERSISTENT coughing, and thick mucus. If you have chronic lung disease, these symptoms may be all too familiar. While there are many types of lung disease, the most common are asthma, chronic bronchitis, and emphysema. In each of these diseases there is an obstruction of the airflow in and out of the lungs. Chronic bronchitis and emphysema are often referred to as chronic obstructive pulmonary disease (COPD) or chronic obstructive lung disease (COLD). Although asthma, chronic bronchitis, and emphysema can be described separately, in truth, many patients have a mixture of these diseases and the treatment and self-management approaches often overlap.

Figure 15.1 *Normal Lungs*

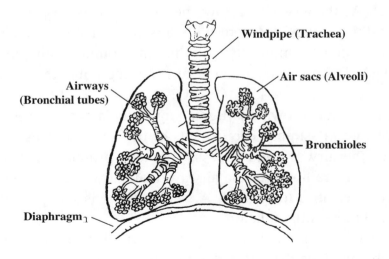

Figure 15.2 *Bronchial Asthma*

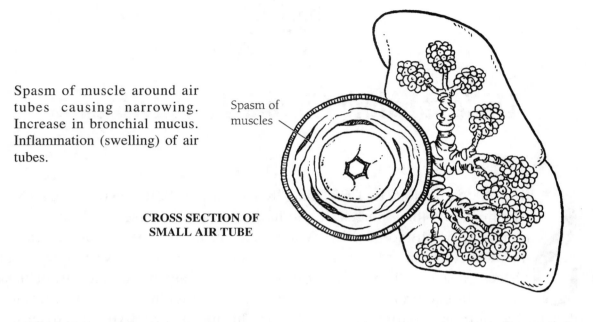

Spasm of muscle around air tubes causing narrowing. Increase in bronchial mucus. Inflammation (swelling) of air tubes.

218

Spasm of muscles

CROSS SECTION OF SMALL AIR TUBE

Understanding Asthma

Our understanding of asthma is changing. Until recently, the focus of attention was on *bronchospasm,* tightening of the muscles of the airways (bronchioles). In asthma, the airways are very sensitive and when exposed to irritants such as smoke, pollens, dusts, or cold air the airways tend to become swollen and narrow (see Figure 15.2). As the airways narrow, the flow of air is obstructed or blocked producing an "asthma attack" or flare with shortness of breath, coughing, chest tightness, and wheezing (a high-pitched whistling sound as air pushes through narrowed airways). Treatment is aimed at relaxing the temporarily tightened airway muscles.

However, research has shown that tightening of the airways (bronchospasm) is not the whole picture in asthma. The irritants or triggers also cause *inflammation* with swelling of the airways and excessive mucus production. Chemicals are released from the surface lining of the airways that cause the inflamed airways to become even more sensitive to irritants. A vicious circle is set up, leading to more bronchospasm and more inflammation.

Therefore, it is often not enough to treat the acute flare of bronchospasm with bronchodilator medications that relax the muscles in the airways. Effective treat-

Figure 15.3 *Chronic Bronchitis*

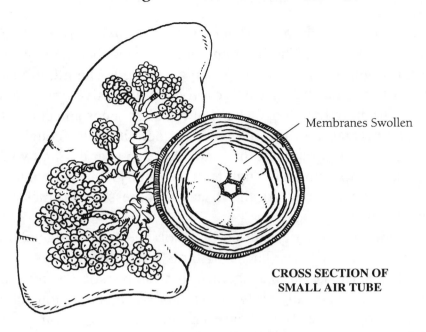

Membranes Swollen

CROSS SECTION OF SMALL AIR TUBE

Inflammation causing narrowing of air tubes and increase in bronchial mucus.

ment involves *avoiding irritants* in the environment and the use of anti-inflammatory medications such as corticosteroids or cromolyn to reduce the swelling, inflammation, and excessive reactivity of the airways. Environmental control strategies and anti-inflammatory medications must be used even when you are not feeling any symptoms in order to help *prevent* acute attacks. Avoiding smoking and secondhand smoke is especially important for people with asthma.

Asthma varies dramatically from person to person. Symptoms may consist of mild wheezing or shortness of breath at night (asthma symptoms tend to be worse during sleep). The attacks may be mild and infrequent. The acute episodes may be severe and life-threatening. For most people, asthma can be effectively managed. But your involvement as an active partner in care is essential. You can learn to avoid triggers that make symptoms worse and monitor lung function and take action to prevent symptoms and acute attacks. You can develop a plan with your doctor to recognize and effectively treat symptoms. You can also learn how to breathe effectively and exercise properly. While these measures cannot completely cure or reverse the disease, they can help you reduce symptoms and live a full, active life. By taking an active role in self-management, you should be able to participate fully in work and leisure activities, sleep through the night without coughing or wheezing, and avoid emergency visits to the doctor and hospitalizations for asthma.

Understanding Chronic Bronchitis

Chronic bronchitis is a chronic *inflammation and thickening of the lining of the airways* (bronchial tubes). The inflammation narrows the opening of the airways and interferes with the flow of air (see Figure 15.3). The inflammation also causes the glands that line the airways to produce excessive amounts of thick mucus, further obstructing breathing. The result is often a chronic cough that produces mucus (sputum) and shortness of breath. By definition, the cough in chronic bronchitis must be present for at least three months each year during two consecutive years. At first, the sputum and cough tend to occur just in the winter months, but soon may occur year round. As the disease progresses, shortness of breath may become more severe.

Chronic bronchitis is primarily caused by smoking. Air pollutants, dusts, and toxic fumes can also contribute. These irritants keep the airways continually inflamed and swollen. The key to management is to stop smoking and avoid other irritants. If this is done, especially early in the disease, the condition can often be prevented from getting worse. If you have chronic bronchitis, you should get a *yearly influenza (flu) vaccine and a once-in-a-lifetime pneumoccal pneumonia vaccine.* Also, avoid exposure to anyone with a cold or influenza. These infections can greatly aggravate the symptoms of bronchitis. Your doctor may also recommend the use of medications to *thin and liquefy mucus* as well as occasional treatment with *antibiotics* if symptoms get worse (increased cough with yellow-brown sputum, increased shortness of breath, and/or fever). Some of the medications that might be prescribed are discussed in more detail later in this chapter.

Understanding Emphysema

In emphysema, the tiny air sacs *(alveoli)* at the very ends of the airways are damaged (see Figure 15.4). The air sacs lose their natural elasticity, become overstretched, and often break. The damaged air sacs are less able to bring fresh oxygen into the bloodstream and to get rid of carbon dioxide wastes. The tiniest airways also narrow, lose their elasticity, and tend to collapse during exhalation. The stale air gets trapped in the air sacs and fresh air cannot be brought in.

A significant amount of lung tissue can be destroyed before symptoms appear. This is because most of us have a large reserve of lung capacity. However, at a certain point, the lung capacity is diminished to the point where the patient begins to notice shortness of breath with exertion and physical activity. As the disease progresses, the shortness of breath becomes worse with less exertion and eventually may be present even when at rest. A cough producing mucus may also occur.

Figure 15.4 *Emphysema*

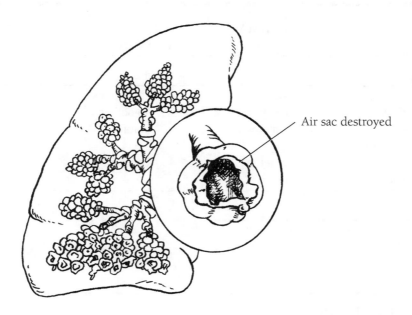

Air sac destroyed

Enlarged and destroyed air sacs causing big air spaces in the lung tissue.

Smoking is the major cause of emphysema. While cigarette smoking is the most common and dangerous cause, cigar and pipe smoking are also damaging. Even if you do not smoke, daily exposure to passive, or "secondhand," smoke is almost as bad. It is important that your home, car, and workplace are smoke-free. There is also a rare hereditary type of emphysema caused by an inherited deficiency of an enzyme that normally protects the elastic tissue in the lungs. Emphysema tends to get progressively worse, especially if smoking continues. The key to prevention and treatment is avoiding all smoking. Although quitting smoking sooner rather than later is better, quitting at any stage of the disease can help preserve remaining lung function. Patients with emphysema can learn a variety of self-management strategies, from proper breathing to efficient exercise to maximize the ability to lead an active life. Medications and oxygen can sometimes be helpful in emphysema as described below.

Asthma, chronic bronchitis, and emphysema most often overlap, so you may have one or more of them. While the treatment varies somewhat depending on the specific symptoms and disease, some of the principles and strategies of management are similar (see Table 15.1, "Chronic Lung Disease at a Glance"). In addition to the self-management strategies described throughout this book, let's take a closer look at some of the management approaches specific to chronic lung disease.

Table 15.1 *Chronic Lung Disease at a Glance*

	ASTHMA	CHRONIC BRONCHITIS	EMPHYSEMA
FEATURES			
Sensitivity to triggers	common	sometimes	no
Spasm of airways	common	sometimes	sometimes
Inflammation *(swelling)* of airways	common	common	rare
Excess mucus	sometimes	common	sometimes
Damaged air sacs	no	no	common
SYMPTOMS			
Cough	common	common	sometimes
Shortness of breath	sometimes	sometimes	common
Wheezing	common	sometimes	sometimes
Mucus	sometimes	common	sometimes
PROGNOSIS (OUTLOOK)			
	symptoms almost always controllable with treatment	early disease may be reversible, but advanced disease may progress	damage is permanent, but progression may be slowed
PREVENTION			
Avoid triggers	important, especially smoking	important, especially smoking	important, especially smoking
Immunizations	influenza (annual) pneumonia (once)	influenza (annual) pneumonia (once)	influenza (annual) pneumonia (once)
TREATMENT			
Bronchodilators:			
Adrenaline-like	common	sometimes	sometimes
Theophylline	sometimes	sometimes	sometimes
Ipratropium	sometimes	common	common
Anti-inflammatory:			
Steroids	common	sometimes	sometimes
Cromolyn sodium	common	never	never
Expectorants/Mucolytics	rare	sometimes	sometimes
Antibiotics	rare	common	sometimes
Oxygen	rare	sometimes	common
Breathing exercises	sometimes	common	common

Avoiding Irritants and Triggers

The best way to manage chronic lung disease is to avoid the things that make it worse. Several types of irritants can trigger the symptoms of asthma and worsen the symptoms of other types of chronic lung disease. Fortunately, you can learn to eliminate or avoid many of the irritants and, when that isn't possible, at least gain control over others.

Smoking

Whether you smoke yourself or are around people who smoke, smoking irritates and damages the lungs. The hot smoke dries, inflames, and narrows the airways. The poisonous gases paralyze the cilia, the tiny hairlike sweepers in your airways that help clean out dirt and mucus. The carbon monoxide in cigarette smoke robs your blood of oxygen and makes you feel tired and short of breath. The irritation from smoking makes infections more likely and can irreversibly destroy the air sacs deep in the lungs. *Smoking is the principal cause of chronic bronchitis and emphysema and a major trigger of asthma.* The good news is that most of these harmful effects can be eliminated by quitting smoking and by avoiding secondhand smoke.

Air Pollution

Dirt and fumes added to the air, whether from automobile exhaust, industrial wastes, household products, aerosol sprays, or wood smoke from fireplaces, can irritate sensitive airways. On particularly smoggy days, check your radio and TV for air pollution alerts and try to stay indoors as much as possible.

Cold Weather

For some people, very cold air can irritate the airways. If you can't avoid the cold air, try breathing through a cold-weather mask (available at most drugstores) or a scarf.

Allergens

An allergen is anything that triggers an allergic reaction. If you have asthma, an attack may be triggered by both outdoor and indoor allergens. Avoiding allergens completely can become a full-time job. Still, a few sensible measures significantly reduce exposure. When pollen and mold spore counts are high, it's best to stay indoors in an air-conditioned environment.

For some people, however, the major allergic triggers are found indoors in the form of house-dust mites, animal hair (dander), and molds. Often pet dogs, cats, and birds have to be banished from the house or at least from bedrooms if a person reacts to pet allergens. Bathe dogs and cats weekly to reduce allergens. House-dust mites tend to live in mattresses, pillows, carpets, upholstered furniture, and clothing. At a minimum, an allergic person should cover the mattress and pillows with airtight covers, wash bedding weekly, avoid sleeping or lying on upholstered furniture, remove carpets from the bedroom, and, if possible, avoid dusting and vacuuming. Damp mopping is recommended rather than dusting or vacuuming, which can scatter allergens in the air. Also, change heating and air-conditioning filters each month. It may take some time and repeated cleaning to rid the environment of harmful levels of pet, mite, or dust allergens.

Household products like perfumes, room deodorizers, fresh paint, and certain cleaning products can also trigger asthma symptoms in susceptible people. For some people, indoor air cleaners can also be helpful in reducing allergens in the air. For some people with asthma, allergy testing can help identify specific allergic triggers and "allergy shots" (immunotherapy) may help desensitize a person to certain allergens. Certain foods (e.g., peanuts, beans, nuts, eggs, shellfish, and milk products) and food additives (e.g., sulfites in wine and dried apricots) can also trigger asthma symptoms in some people.

Medications

Certain medications can cause wheezing, shortness of breath, and coughing in some people. These include anti-inflammatory medications like aspirin, ibuprofen, and naproxen, as well as beta-blockers (such as propranolol) used to treat high blood pressure and heart disease.

Infections

Colds, influenza, sinus infections, and infections of the airways and lungs can make breathing more difficult for those with chronic lung problems. While you can't prevent all infections, you can reduce your risks. Make sure to get an influenza immunization (flu shot) each year in the early fall and a one-time vaccine for pneumococcal pneumonia. Try to avoid people with colds. To cut down on the spread of viruses, wash your hands frequently and don't rub your nose and eyes. Also, discuss with your doctor how to adjust your medications if you get an infection. Early treatment can often prevent serious illness and hospitalizations.

Exercise

Exercise can be a problem and a benefit for people with chronic lung disease. On one hand, physical activity can improve strength and enhance the capacity of the heart and lungs. On the other hand, vigorous physical exercise can trigger asthma symptoms and cause uncomfortable shortness of breath in people with chronic lung disease. There are ways to choose exercise routines (see Chapters 6 through 9) and adjust your medications before exercising to prevent exercise-induced asthma. If being able to exercise comfortably is a problem, discuss this with your physician.

225

Emotional Stress

Emotional stress does not cause chronic lung disease. However, it can make the symptoms worse by causing the airways to tighten and breathing to become rapid and shallow. Many of the breathing and relaxation exercises in this book can help prevent the worsening of symptoms. Also, learning how to manage your disease helps you feel more in control and less stressed in general.

The effect of triggers can be additive. For example, your cat alone may not trigger an acute attack, but if you add a cold, cleaning chemicals, or stress, then an attack may occur.

Self-Monitoring Lung Function

For people with asthma and even patients with emphysema or COPD, the measurement of lung function at home can be a life-saver. The symptoms of wheezing, shortness of breath, and coughing are not always good indicators of the severity of asthma or the response to medications. You can, however, learn a simple, at-home technique to more accurately measure your lung function. You'll need a *peak flow meter,* which is a pocket-sized instrument costing $15–30. With the aid of this device, you can accurately measure how quickly you can blow the air out of your lungs. Peak flow rates are an early warning system to alert you that trouble is building up even hours or days before you experience any increase in coughing, wheezing, or chest tightness. Lower-than-usual peak flow rates may mean that the airways are constricted, inflamed, and obstructed. Knowing your airways are closing down can allow you to take action and adjust your medications before symptoms flare. Peak flow rates as high as your "personal best" or as high as those predicted for a healthy person your age, sex, and height, tell you that your asthma is under control.

If you have moderate or severe asthma, the peak flow meter can become a best friend. It can be a very helpful tool for safe and effective asthma self-management by alerting you to problems before they become severe. It can help you and your doctor know when medications need to be increased and when they can be safely tapered. It can help you identify possible allergens or triggers by monitoring your peak flow rates before and after exposure to a suspected agent, environment, or activity. It can help you distinguish between worsening asthma or breathlessness caused by anxiety or hyperventilation. Most of all, it can help you manage your asthma better.

Ideally your peak flow should be checked twice a day to get the earliest clue to an asthma attack or flare. At a minimum, check your peak flow once a week when you are well. By checking the peak flow when you are well, you will be able to see how far the peak flow has dropped when you are sick. Be sure to check your peak flow at least twice daily if you get a cold or have a runny nose, coughing, or wheezing. Always check your peak flow *before* taking medications.

How to Use a Peak Flow Meter

General instructions are given below, but please follow the specific instructions that come with your meter or are given by your doctor, nurse, or respiratory therapist.

1. Move the marker to zero or the lowest number on the scale.
2. Stand up and take as deep a breath as you can.
3. Place the meter in your mouth and close your lips tightly around the mouthpiece.
4. **Blow out as hard and fast as possible.** It is extremely important that you make the strongest blast of air you possibly can.
5. Write down the number indicated.
6. Repeat the process two more times.
7. Record the **highest** of the three numbers achieved.

Asthma Self-Management Plan

Work out a plan with your doctor about what specific actions you should take based on your peak flow measurements (see sample Asthma Self-Management Plan). For example, if your peak flow reading drops to 50–70% of your personal best or predicted measurements, your doctor may instruct you to increase your inhaled bronchodilator medications or perhaps start a steroid medication. You'll need to work out an individual plan of action with your doctor. If you wait until your symptoms get worse, they will be more difficult to treat. Early action and adjustment of your medications can make a critical difference.

Asthma Self-Management Plan (Adults)

Name:	MR#:	Date:	MD:	MD Office Phone:

- Use of your daily peak flow/symptom diary will give you better control of your asthma.
- MY PERSONAL BEST PEAK FLOW READING = _____.
- If your peak flow is less than 80% of your personal best, check your peak flow 2–3 TIMES A DAY and follow the self-management plan on this page and the next as indicated.
- Always **use a spacer with your inhalers.**
- At the **start** of a **cold**, follow your SELF-MANAGEMENT PLAN in the YELLOW ZONE and monitor your peak flow carefully.
- During your **"asthma season,"** monitor your peak flow carefully and anticipate the need to step up to your YELLOW ZONE plan.

GREEN ZONE

THIS IS YOUR DAILY PLAN.

ABOVE 80% _____ (OPTIMALLY 90%_____)

Able to do usual activities.

Sleeping all night

Your asthma bothers you less than twice a week.

ACTION

Controller: Azmacort®/Flovent®/Pulmicort® _____ puffs _____ times/day.

Reliever: Albuterol®: **Take only if needed** for asthma symptoms.

　　　　　2 or ___ puffs 20 min. before exercise or every ___ hours as needed for asthma symptoms.

(Your reliever should NOT be used regularly when you are in the green zone.)

Other: _____ mg or puffs every ___ hours or ___ times/day.

Other: _____ mg or puffs every ___ hours or ___ times/day.

YELLOW ZONE

INCREASE IN SYMPTOMS. Also use at the **start of a cold** and continue for _____ days afterward. Range 50% _____ to 80% _____.

Increased asthma symptoms—including waking at night.

Usual activities somewhat limited.

Increased cough, chest tightness, or wheezing.

Peak flow does not return to the green zone after a few doses of the bronchodilator.

ACTION

Consider what may be causing your flare-up (e.g., infection, heartburn, allergies, smoke, etc.) and treat the problem.

Increase fluid intake.

Increase Controller:　Azmacort®/Flovent®/Pulmicort® to ___ puffs ___ times/day.

Increase Reliever:　Albuterol® to___ puffs every ___ hours until back into green zone

　　　　　　　　　Then use as needed.

Other: _____ mg or puffs every ___ hours or ___ times/day. (Same as green zone)

Other: _____ mg or puffs every ___ hours or ___ times/day. (Same as green zone)

If you are not improving after 2–3 days and your Peak Flow remains below 65% _____, use the Yellow Zone controller dose for at least 2–3 weeks and begin Prednisone/Medrol® dose as in the red zone. CALL THE NUMBER AT THE TOP OF THIS FORM OR _____.

227

(continues)

Asthma Self-Management Plan (Adults)
(continued)

RED ZONE

MEDICAL ALERT.

BELOW 50% _____ **before** Reliever

Asthma medications have not reduced symptoms.

Peak flow reading stays low.

Very short of breath.

Usual activities severely limited.

Persistent cough, wheeze, and/or waking up several times at night due to asthma.

ACTION

Immediately begin Prednisone/Medrol® dose _____ mg _____ times daily.

Increase Reliever: Albuterol® 4–6 puffs or nebulizer every 10–20 minutes up to 3 times only.

                        Then _____ puffs every ____ hours.

Controller: Azmacort®/Flovent®/Pulmicort® ___ puffs ___ times/day.

Other: _____ mg or puffs every _____ hours or _____ times/day. (Same as green zone)

Other: _____ mg or puffs every _____ hours or _____ times/day. (Same as green zone)

CALL THE NUMBER AT THE TOP OF THE FORM (PREVIOUS PAGE) OR _____.

If not significantly improved, go to the EMERGENCY ROOM.

Have a plan for getting Emergency Care QUICKLY.

ALWAYS CARRY A RELIEVER MEDICATION WITH YOU.

DANGER SIGNS:

Difficulty walking/talking due to shortness of breath.

Unable to catch breath or struggling to breathe.

GO TO THE EMERGENCY ROOM OR CALL 911 NOW.

© Kaiser Permanente Medical Care Program. Reprinted with permission.

Medications

Effective management of chronic lung disease often involves a combination of medications. Bronchodilator medications are designed to relax the muscles surrounding the airways and open the airways wider. Inhaled bronchodilators work within minutes to relieve the wheezing and shortness of breath. Anti-inflammatory medications may also be prescribed to reduce the inflammation, swelling, and reactivity of the airways. For those with chronic bronchitis and emphysema, medications to loosen mucus (mucolytics and expectorants) as well as antibiotics may be used.

Some of the medications may be used to relieve symptoms such as wheezing, while others may be used to prevent symptoms. Some medications may be used to both treat and prevent. When the medications are being used to prevent symptoms, they must be taken regularly, even when symptoms are not present. Too often people stop their medications because they feel better. Discuss with your doctor which medications to continue and which may be stopped as symptoms improve.

Some people worry that they will become addicted to the medications or that they may become "immune" and no longer respond to the medication. *None of the medications used to treat lung disease are addictive. Nor do patients become "immune" to the medications.* If your medications are not working well to control your symptoms, discuss this with your doctor so that adjustments can be made.

229

Bronchodilator Medications

Adrenaline-like Medications (Beta-Adrenergic Agonists)

Examples: albuterol (Proventil, Ventolin), pirbuterol (Maxair), metaproterenol (Alupent, Metaprel), terbutaline (Brethine, Bricanyl), salmeterol (Serevent)

How They Work: These medications are similar to adrenaline (epinephrine), a substance produced in the body. They stimulate tiny nerve receptors in the smooth muscles that surround the airways and cause the muscles to relax, rapidly reversing the bronchospasm, opening the airways, and making breathing easier. These medications are most often inhaled, but some can also be taken orally (pills or liquids). In the emergency room or hospital, they may be given intravenously or by injection.

Possible Side Effects: Shakiness, tremor, nervousness, restlessness, irregular or increased heart rate, insomnia, nausea, headache. The side effects tend to be less with inhaled medications than with the oral form of the medications.

Comments: The inhaled form takes only a minute or two to begin working while the oral form may require more than 30 minutes to start relieving symptoms (see "Steps for Using an Inhaler" on page 235). These medications may be used regularly to help prevent asthma symptoms or on an "as needed" basis to treat suddenly worsening symptoms. It is usually easier and takes less medication to prevent symptoms or to stop an episode in its early phase than later. Always carry an inhaled bronchodilator with you so that it is available at the first sign of increasing symptoms. Inhaled bronchodilators can also be used 5 to 15 minutes before exercising by people who tend to develop wheezing during or after exercise. While the bronchodilator medications can help quickly relieve the muscle tightness and associated narrowing of the airways, they do not treat the underlying inflammation. Therefore, if you are having to use the inhaled brochodilator often (twice a week or more), discuss this with your doctor. You may need an additional anti-inflammatory medication.

Theophylline

Examples: aminophylline (Slophyllin, Somophyllin, Slobid, Theo-Dur, Resbid, Theolair-SR, etc.)

How It Works: This medication relaxes the muscles surrounding the airways to reduce wheezing and shortness of breath. It can be used to treat an asthma attack or on a regular basis to prevent airway constriction. The medication can be given intravenously (I.V.) in the hospital or taken orally as a pill or liquid. The oral forms of the medication take 45 minutes or more to begin working.

Possible Side Effects: Stomach upset (heartburn and nausea), diarrhea, irritability, headache, dizziness, shakiness, insomnia, nervousness, frequent urination, difficulty urinating (especially in men with prostate-gland enlargement), rapid or irregular heartbeat, and, rarely, seizures. Taking the medication with meals can help reduce the stomach irritation.

Comments: Your doctor may order blood tests to measure the levels of theophylline in your blood. If it is too low, it may not be effective. If it is too high, it may be toxic. The usual therapeutic range is 5–20 mcg/mL. Theophylline is prescribed somewhat less frequently today because of the more widespread use of the beta-adrenergic bronchodilators and corticosteroid medications. Theophylline may be used in combination with these other medications. The long-acting forms of theophylline are convenient (taken only twice a day) and can be useful in controlling nighttime wheezing in some people.

Ipratropium Bromide

Examples: Atrovent

How It Works: This newer medication blocks constriction of the airways. It is used more commonly to treat emphysema and chronic bronchitis than asthma. It is available in inhaled form.

Possible Side Effects: Dry mouth and throat, cough, headache, nausea, and blurred vision.

Comments: This medication, unlike the adrenaline-like bronchodilators described above that work within minutes, takes longer to open the airways and needs to be used regularly to be maximally effective.

Anti-Inflammatory Medications (Symptom Preventers)

Cromolyn Sodium

231

Examples: Intal

How It Works: This inhaled medication prevents asthma attacks by inhibiting the release of chemicals in the airways that cause inflammation, allergic reactions, and narrowing of the airways. Since it has an anti-inflammatory effect and is used to prevent asthma attacks, it should be used regularly, not just when symptoms worsen. It can also be used to prevent symptoms that occur from exercise or allergens (such as pets or pollens), if it is used 5 to 60 minutes before contact.

Possible Side Effects: Cough

Comments: It is difficult to predict which people will benefit from cromolyn. You may need to use the medication for a full 4 to 6 weeks before you know how well it will work for you. If you are taking an inhaled bronchodilator as well as inhaled cromolyn, use the bronchodilator first and wait 5 minutes before using the cromolyn. This increases the amount of cromolyn reaching the smaller airways.

Inhaled Corticosteroids

Examples: beclomethasone (Beclovent, Vanceril), triamcinolone (Azmacort), flunisolide (Aerobid), fluticasone propionate (Flovent)

How They Work: These medications gradually decrease inflammation, swelling, and spasm of the airways and prevent overreaction of airways to asthma triggers like allergens. You may have to take the inhaled steroid medication for 1 to 4 weeks to see its full benefit. The inhaled steroids are now being recommended for use more often in patients with recurrent or moderately severe symptoms. Since inhaled steroids are not rapid acting, they are not helpful in the immediate treatment of a severe asthma attack.

Possible Side Effects: Coughing, hoarseness, and yeast (candida) infections in the mouth. The risk of irritation and infection can be greatly reduced by using a spacer or holding chamber (see page 236) and by rinsing excess medication out of your mouth after inhaling. Because only small amounts of inhaled steroids reach the bloodstream, they tend to have fewer and less serious side effects than does long-term use of oral steroids (see below). (Note: The corticosteroid medications used to treat asthma are completely different from the anabolic steroids sometimes taken illegally by athletes.)

232

Comments: If you are taking an inhaled bronchodilator as well as an inhaled steroid, use the bronchodilator first and wait 5 minutes before using the inhaled steroid medication. This increases the amount of steroid medication reaching the smaller airways.

Systemic Corticosteroids

Examples: prednisone, dexamethasone (Decadron), methylprednisolone (Medrol), triamcinolone (Aristocort)

How They Work: The corticosteroids or steroid medications work gradually to both prevent and reduce inflammation, swelling and spasm of the airways, and overreaction of the airways to asthma triggers like allergens. They can be taken orally, given intravenously (I.V.), or inhaled. It usually takes several hours for the steroid medications to begin reducing airway inflammation.

Possible Side Effects: With short-term treatment (less than 2 weeks), there appear to be no serious long-term effects, but you may experience slight weight gain, increased appetite, mood swings, fluid retention, and stomach upset. However, long-term steroid treatment with doses above 10 mg per day can result in more serious side effects including stomach ulcers, menstrual irregularities, muscle cramps, acne, thinning of bones (osteoporosis), cataracts, thinning and bruising of the skin, and disruption of adrenal gland function. Stomach upset can be reduced by taking the oral steroid medication along with food. Inhaled steroid medications (see below) have fewer side effects. (The types of corticosteroid medications used to treat asthma are not like the anabolic steroids taken illegally by some athletes, which can have devastating effects on the liver, heart, and muscles.)

Comments: If you are taking oral steroid medications, **do not** suddenly stop taking them. They need to be slowly tapered over days to weeks on a schedule worked out with your doctor.

Expectorants and Mucolytics

Examples: water, guaifenesin, potassium iodide, acetylcysteine, iodinated glycerol (Organidin)

How They Work: These agents may help make mucus thinner and easier to cough up. Make sure to drink an adequate amount of water to liquefy and thin mucus (6–8 glasses a day).

Possible Side Effects: Varies with the product.

233

Antibiotics

Examples: ampicillin, amoxicillin, Azithromycin, penicillin, erythromycin, tetracycline, sulfa antibiotics (Septra, Bactrim), cephalosporins, quinolones

How They Work: Antibiotics help the body fight bacterial infections. People with chronic lung disease are prone to develop bacterial infections of the airways (bronchitis) or the lungs (pneumonia).

Possible Side Effects: These vary with the specific antibiotic but sometimes include nausea, vomiting, and diarrhea. Rashes, increased difficulty breathing, or fever may indicate a more serious allergic reaction, and the antibiotic should be stopped until a doctor is consulted.

Comments: Always take your antibiotic for the full time prescribed (usually 5–10 days or longer) even though you feel better. If you stop too soon, the infection may recur. Follow the instructions with each antibiotic. For example, tetracycline should not be taken with any milk products or antacids, since they interfere with the absorption of the drug and reduce its effectiveness.

Inhalation Treatments

Metered-Dose Inhaler (MDI)

Some lung medications such as bronchodilators, corticosteroids, and cromolyn can be taken by inhalation. They come in a special canister called a metered-dose inhaler (MDI). When used properly, inhalers can be a highly effective way of quickly delivering medication to your lungs. By breathing medicine directly into the lungs instead of swallowing it in a pill form, you absorb less medication into the bloodstream causing fewer side effects while allowing higher concentrations of medicine to reach the lungs.

However, learning to use an inhaler properly is more difficult than swallowing a pill. It takes proper instruction and some practice. The instructions given below are good as background information, but *it is essential to have a health professional knowledgeable about inhaler use observe you periodically to check your technique. Improper use of inhalers is one of the most important reasons for failure to control symptoms. So, if you are prescribed an inhaler, make sure to get help in using it properly.*

Which Inhaler Should I Use First?

If you are taking two inhaled medications, use the quick-acting symptom-relieving (bronchodilator) medication first. Wait several minutes for it to open up the breathing tubes so that the preventive (inhaled anti-inflammatory) medication can get into your lungs better.

How to Check If Your Inhaler Is Full or Nearly Empty

An inhaler may discharge or spray even when there is no medicine left. To find out if your inhaler has any puffs of medication left, use one or more of these methods:

1. The canisters usually say the number of puffs they contain when new. Divide the number of puffs in the canister by the average number of puffs you use each day. This will give you the approximate number of days the medication will last. Mark this day on your calendar or the inhaler. When the day comes, consider the inhaler to be empty.

2. Make a check mark each time you take a puff. When the number of check marks equals the number of puffs in your inhaler, your inhaler is empty.

3. Some inhalers will float to the surface of a bowl of water when they are empty and sink when they are full (see Figure 15.5). Test the canister without the plastic mouthpiece. This method works with most inhalers but not with cromolyn (Intal), nedocromil (Tilade), and Aerobid inhalers.

Figure 15.5 *Checking Your Inhaler*

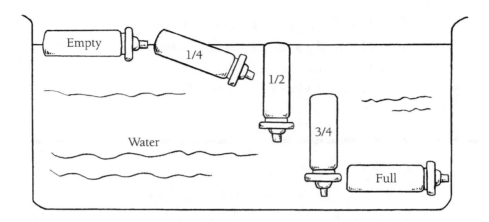

Steps for Using an Inhaler*

1. Shake the inhaler up and down several times (about 5 seconds).

2. Remove the cap on the mouthpiece and hold the canister upright with your thumb supporting the bottom and index and middle fingers on top. Position the mouthpiece 1–2 inches in front of your mouth (or see the instructions on page 236 for using a spacer).

3. Open your mouth wide, tilt your head back slightly, and breathe out fully.

4. Now begin to breathe in ***slowly*** as you press down on the canister to release a spray of the medication toward the back of your throat.

5. Breathe in ***slowly and deeply*** for 3–5 seconds.

6. Hold your breath for 5–10 seconds, if possible, to allow the medication to reach deeply into your lungs. Then exhale.

7. Repeat puffs as directed. With bronchodilators, waiting at least 1–2 minutes (5–10 minutes is even better) between puffs may permit the second puff to reach smaller airways better.

8. Rinse out your mouth with water and spit it out, especially if you are inhaling the steroid medications.

---

* We recommend using a spacer with inhaled medications (see below).

Common Errors to Avoid When Using an Inhaler

- Forgetting to shake the canister
- Holding the inhaler upside down
- Breathing through your nose
- Failing to hold your breath
- Inhaling too fast

Spacers or Holding Chambers

To make using an inhaler easier, safer, and more effective, we strongly recommend using a spacer device or holding chamber. This is a chamber (usually a specially designed tube or bag) into which you spray the medication from the inhaler. You then inhale the medication from the spacer. The spacer makes it more likely that you can inhale the smaller, lighter droplets of medication farther into your airways. The spacer also collects on its walls some of the larger, heavier droplets of medication that would otherwise settle in your mouth or throat. This can reduce side effects such as yeast infections in the case of inhaled steroids. Some spacer devices have a whistle that sounds if you are inhaling too rapidly. This also reminds you not to take a fast breath. A fast breath deposits more of the medication in your mouth and less in your lungs.

Spacers are easier to use than metered-dose inhalers alone. You don't have to worry about pointing the spray in the right direction, and your inhalation doesn't have to be as carefully timed and coordinated with the spray. Since more of the medication reaches your lungs and less is left in your mouth with a spacer, the medication tends to be safer and more effective. This is especially important if you are using a steroid inhaler.

Nebulizers

A nebulizer is a device designed to deliver a mist of medicine that you can breathe deeply into your lungs. With some devices, you add the medication and squeeze the bulb to power the spray. Compressor-driven nebulizers have an electric-powered air compressor that forces a stream of air past a solution with dissolved medication. The mist is inhaled through a mouthpiece or mask. The technique for inhaling the medication is similar to that for using metered-dose inhalers.

Oxygen Therapy

For some people with chronic lung disease, their lungs cannot supply the body with enough oxygen from ordinary air. If you are tired and short of breath because there is too little oxygen in your blood, your doctor may order oxygen equipment for you to use at home. Oxygen is a medicine. It is not addicting. Yet some people try not to use it for fear of becoming dependent on it. Supplemental oxygen, however, can provide just the extra boost your body needs to remain comfortable or to perform daily activities without extreme shortness of breath. Some people may require continuous use of oxygen, while others may need oxygen only to help them with certain activities such as exercise.

Oxygen comes in large tanks of compressed gas or small portable tanks of either gas or liquid oxygen. If you are using oxygen, be sure to know the proper dose (flow rates and when to use it and for how long), how to use the equipment, and how to know when to order more. Although your oxygen tank will not explode or burn, oxygen can help other things burn faster. So keep the tank at least 10 feet away from any open flame, including cigarettes.

How to Breathe More Effectively

Breathing Exercises

It is not surprising that breathing is a central concern of people with lung disease. Yet many people find it surprising that proper, effective breathing is a skill that has to be learned. It is not necessarily something that every adult does well naturally. This is especially important for people with lung disease. You can learn some ways to breathe that will enhance the functioning of your respiratory system.

There are two very important breathing exercises: *pursed-lip breathing* and *diaphragmatic or abdominal breathing.* Both help strengthen respiratory muscles (especially the diaphragm) and help rid the lungs of stale, trapped air. One of the primary reasons people with lung disease feel short of breath and can't seem to get enough air in, is because they don't get the old air out. Fresh air can't come in if the lungs are already filled with stale air. These breathing exercises can help you more fully empty your lungs and take advantage of your full lung capacity. (See pages 44–45 for instructions on how to do the breathing exercises).

Posture

If you are slouched over and constricted, it may be very difficult to breathe in and out. Certain body postures make it easier to exhale and inhale fully. For example, if you are sitting, try leaning forward from the hips with a straight back. You can then rest your forearms on your thighs or rest your head, shoulders, and arms on a pillow placed on a table. Or use several pillows at night to make breathing easier.

Clearing Your Lungs

238

Sometimes excess mucus blocks the airways, making it difficult to breathe. Your doctor or respiratory therapist may recommend certain specific positions for "postural drainage." For example, by lying on your left side on a slant with your feet higher than your head, you may be able to help the mucus from certain areas of the lung drain more effectively. Ask your doctor, nurse, or respiratory therapist which, if any, postures would be helpful for you. Also, remember that drinking at least 6 glasses of water a day (unless you have ankle swelling) may help liquefy and loosen the mucus.

Controlled Coughing

A well-executed cough, producing a strong jet of air, is an effective way of clearing mucus from the airways. On the other hand, a weak, hacking, tickle-in-the-throat type of cough can be exhausting, irritating, and frustrating. You can learn to cough from deep in your lungs and put air power into a cough to clear the mucus. Start by sitting in a chair or on the edge of the bed with your feet firmly on the floor. Grasp a pillow firmly against your abdomen with your forearms. Take in several slow, deep belly breaths through your nose and as you exhale fully with pursed lips bend forward slightly and press the pillow into your stomach. On the fourth or fifth breath, slowly bend forward while producing two or three strong coughs without taking any quick breaths between coughs. Repeat the whole sequence several times to clear the mucus.

Exercise Training

Among the simplest and most effective ways to improve your ability to live a full life with chronic lung disease is to exercise. Physical activity strengthens the muscles, improves mood, increases energy level, and enhances the efficiency of the heart and lungs. Although exercise does not reverse the damage to the lungs, it can improve your ability to function within whatever limits you have due to your lung disease. (See Chapter 9 for discussion of physical fitness and exercise for people with chronic lung disease.)

Exercise is good for the heart and lungs. However, some people with asthma may cough or wheeze when they exercise. If you do, you may wish to discuss with your doctor using 2 puffs of albuterol (Ventolin, Proventil) or cromolyn (Intal) 15 to 30 minutes before starting exercise. Wearing a scarf or a mask over your face in cold weather may help prevent the cold air from triggering asthma. Swimming usually does not trigger asthma.

Asthma, chronic bronchitis, and emphysema are by definition not curable. But you can, in partnership with your doctor, work to reduce the symptoms and improve your ability to live a rich, rewarding life.

239

Community Resource Detective's Kit

Chronic Lung Disease Information

American Lung Association, 1740 Broadway, NY, NY 10019-4374, (800) 586-4872

Asthma and Allergy Foundation of America, 1717 Massachusetts Ave., NW, Suite 305, Washington, DC 20036. Hotline 800-7-ASTHMA or (202) 466-7643. www.aafa.org

National Asthma Education Program (NHLBI), P.O. Box 30105, Bethesda, MD 20824-0105, (301) 951-3260.

National Jewish Center for Immunology and Respiratory Medicine, 1400 Jackson St., Denver, CO 80206, (800) 222-5864 for the Lungline. www.njc.org

The Pulmonary Paper, P.O. Box 877, Ormond Beach, FL 32175, (904) 673-5108 for subscription.

• • •

Suggested Further Reading

American Lung Association of Western Pennsylvania. *Self-Help: Your Strategy for Living With COPD.* 3rd ed. Palo, Alto, Calif.: Bull Publishing, 1997.

American Lung Association. *Help Yourself To Better Breathing.* 1991.

American Lung Association. *Around the Clock with COPD.* 1992.

American Lung Association. *The Asthma Handbook.* 1992.

Haas, Francois, and Sheila Spencer Haas. *The Chronic Bronchitis and Emphysema Handbook.* New York: John Wiley & Sons, 1990.

Moser, Kenneth, et al. *Shortness of Breath: A Guide to Better Living and Breathing.* St. Louis, Mo.: C.V. Mosby, 1983.

Petty, Thomas L., and Louise Nett. *Enjoying Life with Emphysema.* Philadelphia: Lea & Febiger, 1987.

Plaut, Thomas. *One Minute Asthma.* Amherst, Mass.: Pedipress, 1992.

16

Understanding Heart Disease and High Blood Pressure

HEART DISEASE AND HIGH BLOOD PRESSURE are among the most common health problems in the developed world. Although there are several types of heart disease, we concentrate on coronary artery disease, which is caused by blockages in the arteries of the heart (the coronary arteries). The blockages themselves are the result of atherosclerosis.

Atherosclerosis develops over a period of several years and is probably initiated by wear and tear damage to the vessel wall due to such factors as high blood pressure, cigarette smoking, high cholesterol, diabetes, and aging (see Table 16.1 for a list of risk factors for heart disease). In response to this damage, cells in the vessel wall and cells in the blood (platelets) begin to multiply and clump together. A tough substance, containing cholesterol and cells from the vessel wall and blood, begins to accumulate on the vessel wall.

When enough of this substance accumulates to reduce the vessel's diameter to less than a third of normal, a condition known as *ischemia* can occur. Ischemia is the lack of sufficient blood supply to the heart muscle. This is dangerous, because the blood flowing through the heart's arteries supplies the heart muscle with the nutrients and oxygen it needs to survive (see Figure 16.1). If a blood clot forms in a narrowed artery, the blood flow and oxygen to the heart muscle can be suddenly stopped, producing a heart attack. Unless the clot is dissolved and blood flow restored quickly, the heart muscle can die.

What Are the Risk Factors for Developing Heart Disease?

Numerous studies over the years have identified several conditions associated with an increased risk for developing atherosclerosis in the coronary arteries. The

Figure 16.1 *The Heart's Arteries*

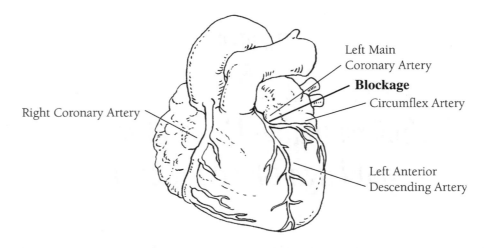

Left Main
Coronary Artery

Blockage

Circumflex Artery

Right Coronary Artery

Left Anterior
Descending Artery

classical risk factors include diabetes, high blood pressure, high cholesterol, cigarette smoking, a family history of premature heart disease (before age 60), being male, and being over age 60. Each "risk factor" by itself can promote the development of heart disease. When a person has more than one of these risk factors, the chance of developing heart disease increases greatly. Fortunately, some of these risk factors are correctable; that is, they can be treated or corrected, so the associated risk of heart disease is reduced. Unfortunately, some risk factors are uncorrectable (see Table 16.1).

High blood pressure, high cholesterol, and cigarette smoking are probably correctable factors. People with high blood pressure or high cholesterol levels can improve these conditions and reduce their risk of heart disease by losing weight (if they're overweight), exercising, and following a healthy diet low in fat and salt.

If those measures fail to normalize blood pressure or cholesterol levels, medications are available to help achieve normal levels. People who smoke can reduce their risk by not smoking. Obesity and physical inactivity are also correctable risk factors that work together to increase risk for heart disease. Diabetes is at least partially correctable. Weight loss, exercise, a prudent low-carbohydrate diet, and medications can help a person with diabetes control her or his blood sugar.

A history of early heart disease of a member of your immediate family (parents, brothers, or sisters) before age 60 appears to identify those people with a genetic predisposition toward developing heart disease. This risk factor is not correctable, at least not with our current level of understanding. Likewise, the increased risk of heart disease that has been associated with men and with people over age 60 does not appear to be correctable.

Table 16.1 *Risk Factors for Heart Disease*	
Potentially Correctable	**Probably Not Correctable**
High Blood Pressure High Cholesterol Cigarette Smoking Diabetes Obesity Physical Inactivity	Family History Male Gender Age Over 60

For many people who already have heart disease, reduction of these so-called cardiac risk factors has been shown to reduce their risk of worsening the disease. For example, several studies have now shown that aggressive lowering of high cholesterol levels can actually *reduce* the amount of atherosclerosis in some people with heart disease. In fact, for most people it's never too late to reduce the risk of developing heart disease or for reducing the risk of worsening existing disease.

What Does Heart Disease Do?

When ischemia occurs, the blood supply is less than the heart muscle requires. The cells of the heart muscle usually weaken and may even die. Your body may let you know that the heart is not getting enough oxygen by giving you the sensation of a squeezing pain or pressure in your chest, commonly known as *angina* or *angina pectoris*. In some people with coronary artery disease, this sensation can radiate from the chest to other parts of the body, including the shoulders, arms, neck, and jaw. The reason angina radiates to other parts of the body is uncertain. It is probably due to the referral of pain along nerve fibers that run close to the heart and go to other parts of the body.

Some people with heart disease experience sweating and nausea. These are usually associated with angina and are probably caused by certain chemicals released by the body in response to stressful events (such as angina). These chemicals may stimulate nerve endings that control sweating and the sensation of nausea.

Other symptoms of coronary artery disease include unusual shortness of breath and fatigue. Shortness of breath and fatigue are probably caused by temporary weakening of the heart during an episode of angina, and results from the lack of proper blood supply to the heart muscle itself. As a result of the shortage of blood, the heart is unable to pump out all the blood it receives. This creates two problems:

- Blood may back up into the lungs, causing shortness of breath,

- The rest of the body will not receive the blood supply it needs, leading to fatigue and further shortness of breath.

When this weakening of the heart is severe and persistent, it is called *heart failure*. Fortunately, not everyone with heart disease experiences heart failure. For those who have episodes of heart failure, treatments are available to improve their symptoms and future outlook (see page 257 for treatment information).

244

Finally, people with heart disease may notice irregular heartbeats. This is caused by irregularities in the conduction system or electrical wiring of the heart. Damage to this system can result in irregular heartbeats, palpitations, skipped beats, or racing beats. Physicians refer to these as arrhythmias or dysrhythmias.

Most irregular heartbeats are minor and not dangerous. However, some forms of arrhythmias can cause problems. Dangerous arrhythmias are often accompanied by episodes of fainting or prolonged irregular heartbeats. Such arrhythmias may be more dangerous for people with severely weakened hearts and those with heart failure. If you notice occasional irregular heartbeats, take note of how frequently they occur, how long they last, how fast your heart is beating (check your pulse), and how you feel during the episode. That information will help your doctor decide whether or not your arrhythmias are dangerous. Remember that infrequent, short bouts of irregular beats are common among many people, both with and without heart disease. They are generally not cause for concern and should not require activity restrictions or treatment with drugs.

Most people with coronary artery disease have at least one of the above symptoms. However, the presence of one of these symptoms does not automatically mean you have heart disease.

In addition, people with heart disease can develop symptoms under varying conditions. For example, one person may develop angina and shortness of breath at the end of a brisk 5-mile walk. Another person may notice those same symptoms at rest. Although both people experienced angina and shortness of breath, the significance of their symptoms is probably not the same. For example, the first person would be able to safely exercise at an intensity below the level that causes his or her angina. The second person, on the other hand, is severely limited by the symptoms and is at high risk for a heart attack.

The same symptoms can represent different levels of concern for different people. The following section will help you identify dangerous symptoms and understand their implications for your future outlook. Remember, if you are ever in doubt about the severity of a symptom you are experiencing, contact your doctor. He or she is your best resource for discussing these issues.

What Is the Outlook for People with Heart Disease?

For people with coronary artery disease, symptoms can come and go. Physical exertion or an emotional upset will sometimes bring on the pain. Most people with such episodes can predict when they are about to happen. That is, they know that a certain amount of exertion or a certain degree of emotional upset will cause symptoms.

Predictable episodes of angina are relatively safe. They can teach you to avoid the levels of exercise or emotional upset that cause angina. If the angina does occur, you can use medicines to relieve the angina and prevent the heart from being overworked.

Unpredictable episodes, on the other hand, may occur at any time for no apparent reason. Because of their unpredictable nature, these episodes are considered to be more dangerous. The underlying cause for all angina is the same: the heart's cells are not getting enough oxygen.

Angina and other symptoms of coronary artery disease are worrisome because they can be associated with one of the most serious outcomes of coronary artery disease—a *myocardial infarction,* or *heart attack.* A heart attack results when the blood supply to an area of the heart is suddenly and completely blocked, leading to heart muscle damage or even death.

For those who survive a heart attack, the severity of heart muscle damage varies from person to person. Generally speaking, the more severe the heart attack, the more heart muscle damage. People with mildly damaged hearts generally do quite well. Some people may have no evidence of ongoing ischemia (the lack of blood supply and oxygen to the heart). Their outlook is very good. Less than 1% of such people have another heart attack the following year.

People with mildly damaged hearts who have episodes of ischemia after their heart attack are at a slightly higher risk of having a future heart attack. Still, only a small number of such people will develop a heart attack during the year following the initial heart attack.

People with severely damaged hearts, on the other hand, are generally at higher risk for subsequent heart attacks. Approximately 10–15% of such people have a heart attack during the subsequent year. In addition, they may develop episodes of heart failure and be physically limited in what they can do. Treatments, including surgical and medical therapies, have been shown to improve the symptoms of heart disease. In many cases, they also improve the long-term outlook, or prognosis, of the disease. (See treatment section on page 257.)

The level of impairment is also somewhat variable, even among people with the same severity of disease. Some people with relatively normal hearts after a heart attack will live relatively normal lives. Others may be limited by the emotional or psychological burdens they feel from having an imperfect heart. They may experience anxiety or depression. They may develop a fear of sexual intimacy. While each person will respond differently, it is important to remember that it is common for people to have worries, anxiety, and even depression. It's also important to remember that these feelings can be helped with improved understanding and control of their disease.

246

With time, a person with heart disease may experience a worsening of symptoms, such as angina (chest discomfort), shortness of breath, or fatigue. Sometimes symptoms will worsen temporarily due to a simple, underlying cause, such as the resumption of cigarette smoking, a change in medications, or suffering an emotionally upsetting experience. At other times, a worsening of symptoms represents a worsening of the coronary artery disease, potentially necessitating more vigorous medical or even surgical therapy.

How can one tell the difference? Call your physician whenever you are concerned about a new symptom. Dangerous symptoms include the development of

- any new chest discomfort,
- unusual shortness of breath,
- dizziness or fainting,
- prolonged irregular heartbeats,
- sudden weight gain,* or
- ankle swelling

What Are the Diagnostic Tests for Heart Disease?

Several tests are helpful in diagnosing heart disease. In addition, these tests help to determine the prognosis, or outlook, for the disease. Exercise testing is one of the easiest and safest tests available. The person usually exercises on a treadmill or a stationary bicycle while hooked up to a monitor of the heart's activities, known as an electrocardiogram. As the intensity of exercise gradually increases, the person is monitored for evidence of ischemia.

The exercise test is particularly useful for people with documented heart disease. It is quite helpful in assessing their prognoses. Following a heart attack, for example, a person without any evidence of ischemia during an exercise test would have a good prognosis.

---

* Patients with congestive heart failure should weigh themselves daily or every other day since weight gain can be the first sign of fluid buildup and an early warning sign the disease is getting worse.

Seek Emergency Care Immediately

If you are having symptoms that might mean a heart attack or stroke, you must seek medical care immediately. New treatments are available that can dissolve blood clots in the blood vessels of the heart and brain and restore blood flow. However, these treatments must be given within hours of the heart attack or stroke—the sooner, the better. In the United States, call 9-1-1 or emergency services if you experience:

Heart Attack Warning Signs
- Severe, crushing, or squeezing chest pain (like someone is sitting on your chest)
- Pain that spreads to the jaw, arms, neck, and/or back
- Pain not relieved by rest or heart medications (nitroglycerin)
- Chest pain occurring with any of the following: rapid and/or irregular heartbeat, sweating, nausea or vomiting, shortness of breath, or light-headedness
- Chest pain that lasts longer than 15 minutes when there is no obvious cause

Stroke Warning Signs
- Weakness, numbness, or paralysis of the face, arm, or leg, especially on only one side of the body, that does not go away in a few minutes
- Blurred or decreased vision in one or both eyes that does not clear with blinking
- Newly developed difficulty speaking or understanding simple statements

Thallium exercise testing is similar to regular exercise testing with one exception. At the end of the monitored exercise session, the person undergoing the test receives an injection of thallium. Thallium is a safe, radioactive chemical that passes through the heart vessels, allowing a special machine to take pictures of the heart. As a result, the thallium exercise test is more accurate at diagnosing heart disease than the regular exercise test. Both are similar in their ability to provide a prognosis.

For those who cannot exercise because of leg or back problems, a special medicine that affects the heart's circulation much like exercise does can be given in lieu of exercise prior to the thallium injection. The thallium test is approximately twice as costly as a regular exercise test.

A *PET scan* is similar to the thallium exercise test, but it does not require a patient to exercise during the test. A PET scan costs about twice as much as a thallium test and is available only in some parts of the country.

Tests measuring how well the heart is pumping can be useful in assessing the prognosis of patients with heart disease (generally, the better it pumps, the better the prognosis). *Ventriculography* is one such test. Using a safe, radioactive chemical injected into a patient's vein, a special machine is able to take a picture of the heart as it pumps and to calculate how well the heart's pumping action is working. Another test is an echocardiogram, a picture created by ultrasound or "sonar" images of the heart as it beats, which measures how well the heart is pumping and how well the heart's valves are opening and closing. Both tests cost approximately the same as a thallium exercise test.

Coronary angiography, or heart catheterization, is an X-ray study of the coronary vessels, considered the "gold standard" of diagnostic studies for the heart. A special dye is injected into the vessels, allowing a clear X-ray image to be taken of the vessels. When no coronary artery disease is present, the image of the vessels is smooth, appearing somewhat like a series of adjoining rivers and streams. When coronary disease is present, however, these images look ragged and sometimes completely blocked off (where the blockages in the arteries are), like a series of dams along a group of rivers and streams. Although this test is the most accurate, it is also the costliest (2–4 times the cost of a thallium test) and most unsafe (approximately 1 patient in a thousand will develop a serious complication, e.g., a heart attack, or may even die during the test).

High Blood Pressure

Blood pressure is a measurement of the amount of pressure in an artery. When the heart contracts, it pushes a wave of blood into the arteries. The systolic pressure is the pressure in the artery when the heart pumps out a wave of blood. The diastolic pressure is the pressure when the heart relaxes between pumps.

The pressures are recorded as millimeters of mercury (mm Hg). When blood pressure is written down, the systolic pressure is always written first followed by a / and then the diastolic pressure. So, a blood pressure of 120/80 means that 120 is the systolic pressure and 80 is the diastolic pressure. Both numbers are important since both high systolic and high diastolic pressures can cause damage.

Hypertension, or "high blood pressure," is often referred to as a "silent" disease. This is because most people with hypertension have no symptoms and cannot tell if their blood pressure is high or not without measuring it. If your hypertension is "silent" and if you feel well, you may find it hard to believe that anything is wrong. High blood pressure (unless it is extremely high) does not usually cause headaches, dizziness, nervousness, fatigue, or pounding of the heart. However, hypertension may not stay silent. Over a period of years, high blood pressure can damage blood vessels throughout the body. In some people, this damage to blood vessels can eventually cause strokes, heart attacks, heart failure, or damage to the eyes and kidneys. The reason for treating high blood pressure is to prevent these complications. *That's why it is important to control your blood pressure even if you don't have any symptoms and feel perfectly well.*

Why do you have hypertension? Over 90% of hypertension is called "primary" or "essential," which really means that the cause is not known.

What is normal blood pressure? A healthy or optimal blood pressure is below 120 systolic and 80 diastolic. Normal is below 130 systolic and 85 diastolic. High normal is between 130 and 139 systolic and between 85 and 89 diastolic. High blood pressure, or hypertension, is considered above 140 systolic and 90 diastolic. As you can see, generally lower is better.

Your blood pressure varies, however, minute by minute. Hypertension is diagnosed when blood pressure measurements are high on two or more occasions. Except in very severe cases, the diagnosis is never based on a single measurement. That's one reason it is important to have repeated measurements of your blood pressure.

One very important self-management skill for those with hypertension is self-measurement of blood pressure. Being able to measure your blood pressure at home or at a drugstore allows you to collect more accurate information about what your blood pressure is throughout the day, not just in the doctor's office. Some people have "whitecoat hypertension" and their blood pressure may be elevated only in the doctor's office and normal at other times. By checking your blood pressure yourself, you can provide additional information to help determine if you do truly have hypertension and, if you do, how well it is responding to lifestyle changes and medications. This will help ensure you are on the lowest possible dosages of antihypertensive medications.

What Is the Role for Lifestyle Changes and Nondrug Treatments?

It is clear from research reports from around the world that lifestyle changes are important for people with heart disease and high blood pressure. The majority of correctable cardiac risk factors can be improved by relatively simple lifestyle improvements.

As mentioned in Chapter 6, developing a consistent and safe exercise program is a cornerstone for developing a healthy lifestyle. Exercise helps to increase vigor and endurance. Coupled with a prudent diet, exercise helps a person achieve and maintain a healthy body weight. Not only can a person's weight improve, but blood pressure, cholesterol, anxiety, and depression can also improve with a program of regular exercise and a healthy eating plan.

A healthy eating plan can be especially helpful in lowering cholesterol and blood pressure. The changes can sometimes be substantial enough to make it possible to not have to use lipid-lowering or antihypertensive medications or to at least lower the dosages. Recent research has shown that an eating plan especially high in fruits and vegetables (8–12 small servings per day) and low-fat or nonfat dairy products (2–4 servings per day) and low in fat can substantially reduce blood pressure. In addition, an eating plan high in calcium, potassium, magnesium, and fiber but low in salt and sodium may help some people reduce blood pressure.

Smoking increases the risk of heart disease and stroke and the chances of getting lung cancer or chronic lung diseases, such as chronic bronchitis and emphysema. Some smokers find it very difficult to quit smoking because the addiction to cigarettes involves not only a physical addiction to nicotine, but also a complex interaction of a smoker's social habits (smoking with friends, for relaxation or pleasure, etc.). The majority of successful quitters do so on their own. They stop buying cigarettes and avoid being around others who smoke. They develop new, healthy habits (walking, singing, chewing on celery sticks, etc.) to help relieve the urge to smoke.

For smokers who find it difficult to quit on their own, many are able to quit with the help of friends, support groups, or health professionals. Nicotine gum or a nicotine patch can be used in some cases to help a person stop smoking. The nicotine in them satisfies the body's craving for nicotine, allowing the person to stop smoking without nicotine withdrawal. Once off cigarettes, the person can then gradually taper down the use of the gum or patch until he or she is completely nicotine-free (and cigarette-free). Additional methods are available to help people who cannot quit smoking on their own. Remember, if you smoke and find it nearly impossible to quit, there are numerous people and resources available to help you.

While low levels of alcohol intake (1 drink per day) may reduce the risk of heart disease, higher alcohol use can increase the risk of both heart disease and hypertension. So, if you do use alcohol, limit the use.

Another important lifestyle skill to learn is relaxation and stress-reduction techniques (see Chapter 5). As mentioned throughout this book, being a self-manager is a key to living well with a chronic illness. Remember that replacing *unhealthy* lifestyle habits with *healthy* ones is one of the most important things you'll do as a self-manager.

What Medications Are Available?

The main medications for heart disease work to improve the heart's blood supply. This can be accomplished in at least two ways:

1. Dilating the blood vessels in the heart, thus improving the blood flow and oxygen supply for the heart muscle itself.
2. Reducing the stress on the heart by slowing the heart rate or improving the efficiency with which the heart muscle contracts.

Some of the medications used for heart disease improve the blood supply to the heart by both of these mechanisms, while others work by only one. The medications most commonly used for heart disease are listed below. There are risks and benefits with all medications. Discuss with your physician how to maximize the benefits and minimize the risks for your particular situation.

Heart and Blood Pressure Medications

Beta-Blocking Agents

Examples: metoprolol (Lopressor, Toprol XL), atenolol (Tenormin), propranolol (Inderal), acebutolol (Sectral), nadolol (Corgard).

How They Work: In general, they lower the work of the heart by lowering blood pressure, slowing the heart rate, and improving the efficiency with which the heart contracts and pumps blood out to the rest of the body.

Possible Side Effects: Sluggishness, dizziness, and depression are experienced by about 15–25% of people on beta-blockers. People with asthma or who experience heart failure find their symptoms worsening while on beta-blockers. Side effects are somewhat less common with some of the newer beta-blockers, such as acebutolol (Sectral), labetolol (Normodyne, Trandate), and pindolol (Visken).

Comments: Beta-blocking agents have been found to improve life expectancy following a heart attack and are commonly used with people with heart disease. If you monitor your exercise intensity by checking your heart rate, beta-blockers will affect your "target heart rate range," since they will lower your maximal heart rate by 10–20 beats per minute. For example, if your target heart rate range is 90–100 beats per minute (23–25 beats per 15 seconds) and you take a beta-blocker, you may notice your heart rate at peak exercise is only 75–80 beats per minute. However, this effect on the heart rate will not necessarily deprive you of significant conditioning available from the exercise. For people on beta-blockers, it may be easier to monitor your exercise intensity by the talk test or perceived exertion methods described in Chapter 8.

Calcium-Channel Blockers

Examples: nifedipine (Procardia XL, Adalat), diltiazem (Cardizem), verapamil (Calan SR, Isoptin SR), nicardipine (Cardene), amlodipine (Norvasc), telodipine (Plendil).

How They Work: They improve angina by dilating the blood vessels, leading to an increased blood supply to the heart muscle itself and reduced blood pressure.

Side Effects: Headache, ankle swelling, dizziness, flushing, and constipation are experienced by 10–20% of people on calcium-channel blockers.

Comments: Nifedipine can increase, while diltiazem and verapamil can reduce your resting heart rate. If you monitor your exercise intensity by checking your heart rate, the calcium-channel blockers may invalidate your "ideal" target heart rate range. Check with your doctor—it may be easier for you to monitor your exercise by using an alternative method, such as the talk test or perceived exertion.

Nitroglycerin

Examples: A pill form (Nitro-bid, Isordil, Dilatrate), a tablet or spray form used under the tongue (Nitrostat, Nitrolingual Spray), and a paste or patch form that is worn on the chest area (Nitro-Dur, Transderm-Nitro, Nitrol Ointment).

How It Works: Nitroglycerin helps improve the blood flow in the heart by improving the efficiency with which the heart pumps out blood, thus reducing the work of the heart. Nitroglycerin appears to dilate the blood vessels in the heart, leading to an increased blood supply to the heart muscle.

Side Effects: Headaches are reported by nearly two-thirds of people who use nitroglycerin. Generally, they are tolerable, especially since they tend to occur only within the first few days of starting nitroglycerin treatment. Other side effects, such as light-headedness and low blood pressure, are experienced by less than 5% of people who use nitroglycerin.

252

Comments: The beneficial effects of nitroglycerin can wear off after several days of continuous use. To avoid such "tolerance," your doctor may have you go several hours each day without your nitroglycerin. This allows the body's tissues to remain sensitive to the effects of nitroglycerin. In addition, nitroglycerin tablets tend to lose their potency over a period of several months, especially if exposed to light and air. You should keep your tablets in an airtight, dark container and obtain a fresh supply every few months to ensure their potency.

Angiotensin Converting Enzyme (ACE) Inhibitors

Examples: captopril (Capoten), enalapril (Vasotec), and lisinopril (Prinivil, Zestril). Several newer agents in this category are currently being developed.

How They Work: ACE inhibitors act by blocking the formation of angiotensin II, an enzyme in the body that causes constriction of blood vessels. The result is that blood vessels are dilated, making it easier for blood to flow through the vessels, and blood pressure is reduced.

Side Effects: Headache, dizziness, and dry cough are occasionally ACE-inhibitor side effects. People taking high doses of these agents can on rare occasions experience a skin rash and the suppression of blood cell production by the bone marrow.

Comments: Although expensive, these agents work well at lowering blood pressure and with few side effects. In addition, they have been found to improve the life expectancy of people with heart failure and help protect against kidney damage in people who have diabetes.

Diuretics

Examples: hydrochlorothiazide (HCTZ, Esidrix), furosemide (Lasix), chlorthalidone (Hygroton), indapamide (Lozol), and triamterene/hydrochlorothiazide (Dyazide, Maxzide).

How They Work: Diuretics, sometimes called "water pills," cause people to eliminate fluid from their bodies by increasing urinary fluid loss. This can lead to a reduction in the amount of fluid in the circulatory system of the body, subsequently reducing the pressure in the blood vessels themselves. Some of these medication also have a direct dilating effect on blood vessels.

Side Effects: Diuretics have a tendency to negatively affect the metabolism of cholesterol, uric acid, and glucose in the blood. Frequent urination, weakness, fatigue, and weight loss are commonly noted. Some diuretics can lead to a low potassium level, a condition that can be dangerous, especially for people with severe arrhythmias. Some diuretics may increase cholesterol, uric acid (may worsen gout), and blood glucose (may interfere with diabetes control).

Comments: Although they are effective at lowering blood pressure and are generally inexpensive, diuretics have been less popular in recent years for blood pressure control. This is due, in part, to side effects. They are probably most effective for people who have had episodes of congestive heart failure, since they help minimize the backup of blood into the lungs and body tissues that someone with a severely weakened heart is at risk for. People taking diuretics should not reduce the amount of fluids they drink.

Other Blood Pressure Medications

Examples: clonidine (Catapres, pill and patch forms), methyldopa (Aldomet), guanabenz (Wytensin), prazosin (Minipress), and hydralazine (Apresoline).

How They Work: Clonidine, methyldopa, and guanabenz act in the brain and the nervous system to prevent vasoconstriction, or tightening, in the blood vessels throughout the body. Prazosin and hydralazine act directly on the blood vessels themselves to cause dilation, or widening, and a subsequent reduction in blood pressure.

Side Effects: Dizziness, drowsiness, dry mouth, depression, headache, and sluggishness.

Comments: These agents are lower in cost than ACE inhibitors and calcium-channel blockers and are fairly effective in lowering elevated blood pressure. Unfortunately, the relatively high frequency of side effects limits their use.

Anti-Arrhythmic Agents

Examples: Numerous agents exist, including lidocaine (Xylocaine), amiodarone (Cordarone), disopyramide (Norpace), encainide (Enkaid), flecainide (Tambocor), mexilitene (Mexitil), procainamide (Procain), quinidine (Quinaglute, Quinadex), and tocainide (Tonocard). Digoxin (Lanoxin), beta-blocking agents, and calcium-channel blockers have some anti-arrhythmic properties and are generally better tolerated than the other agents in this category.

How They Work: The heart has an elaborate system of nerves for conduction of electrical impulses (the "electrical wiring") that allows special "pacemaker" cells

254

in the heart to control the contractions in the four chambers of the heart. These cells fire on a regular, rhythmic basis. Occasionally, these pacemaker cells or the electrical wiring itself become damaged, leading to the irregular firing or conducting of the electrical impulses. The result is an irregular heartbeat or contraction.

In some cases of severely abnormal contractions (such as ventricular tachycardia or ventricular fibrillation), the heart may not pump out an adequate amount of blood to the body, leading to symptoms of ischemia, chest discomfort, shortness of breath, and low blood pressure, for example. Anti-arrhythmic agents work by promoting the proper firing and conduction of each heartbeat. The fact that some of these agents, such as lidocaine, are also used as *topical anesthetics* is an illustration of their stabilizing effects on nerve fibers.

Side Effects: Some agents may lead to fatigue, gastrointestinal complaints (diarrhea, bloating), urinary retention, liver damage, and blood cell disorders (thrombocytopenia, or low platelet levels). Also, all of the agents in this category can potentially worsen the arrhythmias that they are designed to treat.

Comments: The use of anti-arrhythmic agents is generally reserved for life-threatening arrhythmias, since their effectiveness and safety are still somewhat controversial.

Blood-Thinning Agents

Examples: aspirin, and warfarin (Coumadin).

How They Work: Aspirin prevents clotting of the blood by inactivating platelets, blood cells that promote clotting. Warfarin, on the other hand, inhibits vitamin K, a substance that is essential for various steps in blood clotting.

Side Effects: Bruising and bleeding can occur, but are relatively infrequent when these agents are used properly. Aspirin can cause stomach irritation (gastritis) and may even be associated with the formation of a stomach ulcer. High doses of aspirin can lead to ringing in the ears (tinnitus).

Comments: Low-dose aspirin (one-half a tablet every day or every other day) has been shown to reduce the risk of first heart attack. It has also been shown to reduce the risk of recurrent heart attack among those who have had previous heart attacks. Some uncertainty still exists, however, about recommending aspirin because of aspirin's tendency to slightly increase the risk of stroke for people with heart disease. Ironically, aspirin has been shown to reduce the risk of stroke in some studies involving people with atherosclerosis of the arteries in the neck (carotid arteries). Warfarin has been shown to be of benefit in some studies of people with heart disease, but it can also increase the risk of stroke.

The role of these blood-thinning agents is the center of several ongoing research studies, which we hope will shed more light on their health risks and benefits.

Cholesterol-Lowering Agents

Examples: cholestyramine (Questran), colestipol (Colestid), niacin, lovastatin (Mevacor), pravastatin (Pravachol), simvastatin (Zocor), gemfibrozil (Lopid), and probucol (Lorelco).

How They Work: Cholestyramine and colestipol are powders, mixed in water or juice, that bind to bile in the intestine and block bile reabsorption. The liver then uses up cholesterol in the blood to make more bile acids and lowers blood cholesterol. Niacin, statins, gemfibrozil, and probucol lower cholesterol levels by reducing the production of and/or helping eliminate cholesterol in the body (in the liver, in particular, where the majority of cholesterol metabolism occurs).

Side Effects: Cholestyramine can commonly cause heartburn, gas, bloating, or constipation. Niacin can occasionally lead to headache, skin flushing, a skin rash, gout, arrhythmias, heartburn, and even a stomach ulcer. Sustained release forms of niacin have been reported on rare occasion to lead to severe liver damage. Niacin can also increase blood sugar levels of diabetics and uric acid levels of people prone to developing gout. Statins may cause muscle or liver inflammation on very rare occasions, a problem that may necessitate the immediate discontinuation of the medication. Gemfibrozil and probucol are generally well tolerated, with a rare occasion of minor gastrointestinal problems.

Comments: Since many people with heart disease have elevated cholesterol levels, they may be treated with medications if a low-fat diet fails to normalize their cholesterol level. Niacin, a vitamin, is inexpensive and can be effective in normalizing cholesterol levels. Unfortunately, various side effects are common for a large percentage of people using the high doses of niacin required to lower cholesterol levels.

Cholestyramine and colestipol are used as powders and are quite effective at lowering cholesterol levels, although they are among the most expensive agents available for that purpose. Statins are effective, but moderately expensive. Gemfibrozil is effective in normalizing a certain type of blood lipid abnormality, known as hypertriglyceridemia. Probucol is not commonly used for cholesterol control, but is the center of several current studies to measure its risks and benefits for people with abnormal cholesterol levels.

What Procedures Are Available for Treating Heart Disease?

For some people with coronary artery disease, medications alone are not sufficient to improve the blood flow to the heart. For these people, it is necessary to use more "invasive" treatments to improve the limited blood flow. These treatments, sometimes called "revascularization procedures," include balloon angioplasty (technically known as percutaneous transluminal coronary angioplasty or PTCA), and coronary artery bypass surgery. Several newer treatments similar to standard balloon angioplasty are in the developmental stages, such as laser angioplasty and angioplasty, which utilize small "springs" or "stents" in the artery.

In *balloon angioplasty,* a catheter is threaded through the blood vessel containing severe blockage, from a large artery in the arm or leg going to the heart. A very small balloon that surrounds the special catheter is then inflated, breaking up the blockage ("plaque") and widening the opening of the blood vessel. This procedure works fairly well for people with blockages limited to a small area in one or two of the coronary arteries. Up to 30% of people undergoing angioplasty, however, may have a reclosure of the vessels within six months of the procedure, leading to the recurrence of symptoms (angina, shortness of breath, etc.).

Coronary artery bypass surgery is helpful for people with widespread, severe blockages in any or all of their coronary arteries. A blood vessel is taken from either the lower leg or chest wall area and sewn into the diseased vessel(s) of the heart, usually above and below the areas of severe blockage. In this manner, the blood vessel is sewn in as a literal "bypass" for the blood to move around the blocked artery and into the vulnerable area of heart muscle it supplies. Since the surgery involves opening the chest and putting the patient on a "heart-lung machine" (an artificial heart and lung of sorts), risks and complications can be serious. In experienced hands, however, the procedure is not only effective in restoring adequate blood flow to the heart, but is also relatively safe and uncomplicated.

Monitoring Your Progress

As you become familiar with your own particular pattern of symptoms, remember that there may be small fluctuations in their frequency and severity. In those cases where medicines fail to improve your symptoms, stop and ask yourself (and your doctor) what is happening.

257

Could it be that stressful life events have increased recently? Have you changed brands of medicine? Have you changed your diet? Have you begun smoking again? Are you taking a new medicine? Is your pattern of nitroglycerin use causing resistance to its beneficial effects? These and other questions can help in improving your management of your disease. If your physician understands the reasons for your symptoms in these contexts, he/she will be less likely to rush you off to more medicines or bypass surgery and balloon angioplasty. All you may need is some fine-tuning of your current treatment.

Developing healthy lifestyle habits and receiving the medical or surgical treatments that you and your physician decide are right for you can help improve both quality *and* quantity of life.

Summary

Heart disease and high blood pressure affect millions of people each year. Symptoms of heart disease, including angina and shortness of breath, occur when blockages in the heart vessels slow or prevent the flow of blood into the heart muscles. The muscles weaken due to the lack of adequate oxygen and nutrients.

Often the symptoms of heart disease are predictable, such as angina or shortness of breath, after climbing 10 flights of stairs briskly. Some people, however, have more dangerous symptoms—symptoms that come on at unpredictable times. Everyone with heart disease should promptly notify their physician when dangerous symptoms occur. These include new chest discomfort, unusual shortness of breath, dizziness, fainting, prolonged irregular heartbeats, sudden weight gain, and sudden swelling of the ankles.

The outlook for people with heart disease is relatively good for people who are free from ischemia. For those *with* ischemia, the outlook is somewhat poorer and can be estimated by use of various tests available to measure heart function. In addition, their outlook can potentially be improved by the various procedures and medical therapies currently available to patients with heart disease.

• • •

Suggested Further Reading

American Heart Association. *Understanding Angina.* 1984.

American Heart Association. *Exercise and Your Heart.* 1990.

Becker, Gail L. *Heart Smart: A Step-by-Step Guide to Reducing the Risk of Heart Disease.* New York: Simon & Schuster, 1987.

Caplan, Louis R., Mark L. Dyken, and Donald J. Easton. *American Heart Association Family Guide to Stroke Treatment, Recovery and Prevention.* New York: Times Books, 1996.

Evans, Tony (Ed.) *The Stanford Health and Exercise Handbook.* Champaign, Ill.: Leisure Press,1987.

Schoenbert, Jane, and JoAnn Stichman. *Heart Family Hand Book.* Philadelphia, Pa.: Hanley & Belfus, 1990.

Schroeder, John Speer, Tara Coghlin Dickson, and Helen Cassidy Page. *The Stanford Life Plan for a Healthy Heart: The 25 gram Plan Plus 200 Low-Fat Recipes From the World Renowned Stanford University Medical Center.* San Francisco: Chronicle Books, 1997.

Speedling, Edward J. *Heart Attack—The Family Response at Home and in the Hospital.* New York: Tavistock Publications, 1982.

CHAPTER
17

Understanding Arthritis

W HAT IS ARTHRITIS? The word *arthritis* means inflammation of a joint. However, as the word has come to be used, arthritis commonly means virtually any kind of damage to a joint. The most common form of arthritis is *osteoarthritis*. It is the arthritis that generally affects us as we age, causing knobby fingers, swollen knees, or back pain.

Osteoarthritis is not caused by inflammation, although sometimes it may result in inflammation of a joint. The cause of osteoarthritis is not precisely known but involves degeneration or a wearing away of the cartilaginous ends of bone. Because of the degeneration, the bone surfaces become rough and don't move smoothly on one another. Also, the bone ends grow out in the form of spurs (called osteophytes) that create, for instance, the knobs on fingers and heel spurs. Because of these rough surfaces, the lining of the joint is sometimes irritated and makes more than the normal amount of joint fluid. The extra fluid results in swelling.

There are many kinds of arthritis due to inflammation. The most common forms are those caused by rheumatic diseases such as *rheumatoid arthritis* and metabolic diseases such as *gout*. With these diseases, the lining of the joint becomes inflamed and swollen, and also secretes extra fluid. As a result, the joint becomes swollen, warm, red, and tender. If present for a time, *inflammatory arthritis* also results in destruction of cartilage and bone. Such destruction can ultimately lead to deformity. The cause of the inflammation associated with these diseases is not precisely known, but with respect to gout it is clearly related to formation of uric acid crystals in the joint fluid, and in the case of rheumatic diseases it is thought to be due to a form of autoimmunity (an immune or allergic reaction of the body against itself).

Most arthritic diseases do not affect only the joints. Joints are crossed by tendons from nearby muscles that move the joints and by ligaments that stabilize the joints. When the joint lining is inflamed, or the joint is swollen or deformed, those tendons, ligaments, and muscles can be affected. They may become inflamed, swollen, stretched, displaced, thinned out, or even broken. Also, in many places where tendons or muscles move over each other or over bones, there are lubricated surfaces to make the movement easy. These surfaces are called bursae; with arthritis, they too may become inflamed or swollen, causing *bursitis*. Thus, arthritis of any kind does not simply affect the joint. It can affect all of the structures in the region of the joint.

262

What Does Arthritis Do?

From the foregoing discussion, you can see what arthritis does. As a result of irritation, inflammation, swelling, or joint deformity, it causes *pain*. The pain may be present all the time or only sometimes, as when moving the joint. Of all the symptoms of arthritis, pain is the most common.

Arthritis can also *limit motion*. The limitation may be due to pain, to swelling that prevents normal bending, to deformity of the joint or tendons, or to weakness in nearby muscles.

In addition, arthritis can cause problems in areas distant from the arthritis. For example, if the joints of a leg have arthritis, that leg may be favored during walking or other motion. When favoring occurs, posture is often altered and an extra burden is placed on other muscles and joints. *Abnormal posture or extra burdens* can create pain in the affected areas.

One dramatic result of arthritis is *stiffness*. Stiffness of joints and muscles is particularly apparent after periods of rest such as sleeping and sitting. The stiffness makes it difficult to move. However, if you are able to get going, or if you can get heat to the affected joint and muscles (hot pad or hot shower), the stiffness lessens or disappears. For most people, the stiffness lasts only a short while; for an unlucky few, it can last all day. The cause of this stiffness is not clearly known.

Another common consequence of arthritis is *fatigue*. Here, again, the precise cause is not known. Inflammation itself causes fatigue. So does chronic pain, and so does the effort of movement when joints and muscles don't work right. In addition, fatigue is caused by the worries and fears that often accompany arthritis. Whatever its cause, or combination of causes, fatigue is an issue confronting most arthritis patients.

A final consequence of arthritis is *depression.* People with arthritis often have trouble doing what they need or want to do. This can make them feel helpless, angry, and withdrawn, which may lead to depression. Depression can make other symptoms such as pain and disability seem worse. It can reduce an individual's work or social functioning. It can damage family relationships, as well as the capacity for independent living.

Obviously, arthritis can have very damaging effects. In a sense, one might assume that the outlook for a person with chronic arthritis would be bleak. Actually, it is not. Much can be done to offset or eliminate the harmful effects of chronic arthritis. This and related books have been written to describe how that may be achieved. The remainder of this chapter will describe elements of appropriate management, some of which are developed in much greater detail elsewhere in this book.

263

Prognosis, or What Does the Future Hold?

Most arthritic diseases, if left untreated, would have different outcomes for different people. Some would progress more or less steadily to deformity. Others would experience disease that waxed and waned over many years, possibly getting slowly worse but maybe not. A lucky few would have the disease disappear spontaneously. With modern treatment, most patients fall in the last two categories, with far fewer patients proceeding to severe deformity than did years ago.

However, as people live longer without deformity, they also live longer with the various symptoms and problems created by arthritis. That is, they live a life that has been changed in some way by arthritis and, possibly, by the undesirable effects of treatment.

There is no real cure for any of the forms of chronic arthritis. With luck, the arthritis will subside partially or completely on its own. Medical treatment can usually suppress the symptoms and the inflammation, but also must be continued indefinitely. Proper self-management can add greatly to improvement and to prevention of disability. This depends largely on the participation of the person with arthritis and the family. Therefore, prognosis, or what the future holds, cannot be predicted accurately for any individual. It depends in part on medical treatment and on the management program.The future is partly a matter of good fortune, partly in the health professional's hands, and partly in the individual's own hands.

How is Chronic Arthritis Treated?

Drug Treatment

There is no cure for most chronic arthritis. As a result, medical treatment is aimed at preventing or controlling inflammation and pain. The drugs commonly used either help pain or reduce inflammation, or do both. When inflammation is reduced, pain usually declines as a result.

264

Most types of chronic arthritis fluctuate in severity. That is, they get better and worse by themselves. The drugs can speed improvement but they do not cure. Therefore, they must usually be used for long periods of time. The commonly used drugs fall into four categories:

1. *Nonsteroidal anti-inflammatory drugs (NSAIDS).* These drugs have both pain-reduction and anti-inflammatory effects. Of all anti-inflammatory drugs, these are the weakest. They are usually the first drugs used to treat arthritis because they are often helpful and tend to have the least-severe side effects. Representatives of this group include aspirin, Motrin, Indocin, Clinoril, Naprosyn, and Voltaren. In a way, acetaminophen (Tylenol) is also in this group; it reduces pain but has no anti-inflammatory effect. When there is no inflammation involved in the arthritis, as is commonly the case with osteoarthritis, the anti-inflammatory activity of the drug is of no known importance; the benefit is derived from the pain-reducing effect, and therefore aspirin or Tylenol may be as effective as the other NSAIDS.

   Recently, at least two new NSAIDs have been made available, Celebrex and Vioxx. In the pharmacy field, they fall in the COX II inhibitor category. This means that the drugs are designed to have anti-arthritic abilities similar to other NSAIDs but to be less damaging to the stomach and intestines. In practice, the less damaging property may be true, but the anti-arthritic effect is no better than other NSAIDs and may be less. Also, the drugs are expensive. *Potential damage to stomach and intestines by **any** NSAID can be greatly reduced simply by taking the drug in the middle of meals.*

2. *Second line, or "disease-modifying" drugs.* The drugs in this category are all anti-inflammatory drugs, which are more powerful than the NSAIDS but are also potentially more toxic. The term "disease-modifying" is intended to imply healing of inflammatory arthritis,

but healing from these drugs has not been proved. Members of this group of drugs are gold, penicillamine, methotrexate, Azulfidine, Plaquenil, and a new drug, leflunomide (Arava). They are usually used in inflammatory arthritis if NSAIDS fail. They are not used for osteoarthritis.

In recent years, evidence has emerged indicating that earlier use of second-line agents slows the progression of the disease. Because the NSAIDs do not achieve such slowing, many patients with rheumatoid arthritis are receiving treatment with second-line agents early in the course of their disease. Such an early benefit from second-line agents has not yet been shown for other forms of chronic inflammatory arthritis.

3. ***Corticosteroids.*** Corticosteroids are powerful anti-inflammatory drugs that also suppress immune function. Both effects are helpful with inflammatory arthritis, especially for rheumatic diseases in which autoimmune abnormalities appear to play a role in causing the arthritis. Most corticosteroids in use are synthetic versions of a normal human hormone, cortisol, which is present in everybody and exerts a mild masculinizing effect in women. Corticosteroids are the most rapid acting and effective of the antiarthritic drugs, but may cause serious adverse effects when used for long periods of time. Prednisone is the most commonly used corticosteroid. ***One last note: Corticosteroids should never be stopped suddenly.*** Talk with your physician if you are thinking about stopping your use of steroids.

4. ***Cytotoxic drugs.*** These drugs, developed to treat cancer, also have anti-inflammatory and immunosuppressive effects. Examples include Cytoxan, Imuran, Leukeran, and cyclosporine. These drugs can be quite toxic and only sometimes have clear advantages over other anti-arthritic drugs. They are usually used only after other drugs have failed to control the problem. They are never used for osteoarthritis.

5. ***New biological agents.*** Recent evidence has shown that a biological material called "tumor necrosis factor" (TNF) plays an important role in the inflammation of rheumatoid arthritis. TNF is a product of some of the cells involved in the inflammatory and immune responses and is a member of the cytokine family. Two methods of counter-

265

acting TNF have been developed, both of which neutralize TNF. One treatment uses an antibody to TNF called infliximab or Remicade and is still under evaluation. The other treatment method uses a soluble receptor that is obtained from cells to neutralize the TNF. This material is called etanercept or Enbrel. Remicade is given intravenously, and Enbrel is injected subcutaneously. Both drugs have been tested only in rheumatoid arthritis, and both are very expensive.

266

Recently, for osteoarthritis, two unusual therapies have been introduced. Both are intended to improve damaged cartilage or substitute for it. One is glucosamine, taken orally. The other is Hyaluronan, injected into the joint. Studies suggest that glucosamine diminishes symptoms from osteoarthritis in the short-term with a potency similar to low doses of NSAIDs. However, the studies are not definitive and long-term outcomes have not been established. Fortunately, glucosamine appears to have no significant adverse effects. Use of Hyaluronan is more complicated because it requires injections, studies have not demonstrated real benefit to people with arthritis, and the treatment is expensive. Both methods of treatment remain at an early stage of evaluation and appear not to be of decisive benefit to people with osteoarthritis; they have no theoretical or practical value in other forms of arthritis.

At times, other drugs are used. An example is colchicine, which, along with many of the above-mentioned drugs, is effective in treating gout. Antibiotics are used when the arthritis is due to infection.

Only occasionally do the drugs used to treat arthritis provide an immediate benefit. Usually many days or even weeks are necessary before the full effects of the drug are felt. Corticosteroids and colchicine are the exceptions; they can often produce benefit in a matter of hours.

It is almost impossible to predict beforehand whether any of the drugs will be helpful. Therefore, the treatment of chronic arthritis with drugs is a trial and error process, in which the physician usually starts with the mildest medications and proceeds to more powerful drugs if the milder forms fail to benefit the patient.

Most drugs for arthritis are taken by mouth. However, some (corticosteroids, methotrexate, gold, colchicine, Remicade, and Enbrel) can be given by injection into muscles or veins. Injection of corticosteroids directly into inflamed joints can sometimes be very beneficial.

Problems can be caused by the toxic effects of the drugs. All drugs can cause harm as well as benefit. Sometimes a particular drug can be very helpful but also cause so much harm that it cannot be used. Again, it is impossible to predict which drugs will be harmful. With some of the drugs, toxic effects cannot be recognized by the individual and, therefore, the individual must be monitored with blood counts, liver function studies, and/or analyses of urine. People starting on any drug treatment for chronic arthritis should make sure they understand the signs and symptoms of potential harm such as rash, upset stomach, or unusual thoughts, and notify the physician if such symptoms appear.

Sometimes, despite drug treatment, joints are damaged to the point where they cannot be effectively used. Fortunately, today, *surgical techniques* allow for the replacement of many types of joints, and some of the replacement joints function almost as well as natural joints.

267

Some years ago, each type of inflammatory arthritis was treated with a particular group of drugs. Today, almost all of the above drugs are used for any type of inflammatory arthritis. The choice of drugs depends on the person's condition and needs; commonly, milder drugs are used first and more powerful ones are used when milder ones fail. However, as mentioned earlier, stronger drugs are now often used earlier in rheumatoid arthritis in an effort to prevent joint destruction.

Drug treatment is usually helpful. However, it is by no means the only form of treatment. Other forms fall under the general heading of management methods and involve the active participation of the person with arthritis.

Management of Chronic Arthritis

In addition to treatment with drugs or surgery, there are many other ways to achieve good management of chronic arthritis. Certainly as much as for any disease, proper management of arthritis follows the principles outlined in the first two chapters of this book. To understand a complete arthritis management program, it is useful to recall the many consequences of arthritis previously mentioned.

The goal of proper management is not just to avoid pain and reduce inflammation; it is to maintain the maximum possible use of affected joints and the best possible function. This involves maintaining the fullest motion of the joint and the greatest strength in muscles, tendons, and ligaments surrounding the joint. *The key to this goal is exercise.* Exercise, discussed in detail in Chapters 6 through 9, is an essential part of any good management program. The exercise should be regular, consistent, and as vigorous as possible. While exercise may increase pain, it will not make the arthritis worse. In fact, failing to exercise can make arthritis symptoms worse because of physical deconditioning.

Heat is a helpful part of arthritis management. It reduces stiffness and makes movement easier. Many people find that heating joints just before exercise makes the exercise easier. Heat associated with rest can be very soothing. Occasionally, people find cooling of the joint with *ice* to be comforting. Cooling, however, does not increase mobility.

Control of fatigue is important. Rest periods between activities and restful sleep at night are essential for control. When pain disturbs sleep at night, different types of beds (foam beds, water beds) and the use of mild sedation can be of significant help. For some people with arthritis, low doses of anti-depression medication at bedtime will effectively control night pain.

Sometimes, when joint function remains limited, use of assistive devices can be of benefit. Many types of devices are available and are described in the books listed at the end of this chapter.

Altering your eating plan has little value with most types of chronic arthritis, particularly osteoarthritis and rheumatoid arthritis. (What you eat, however, is important for gout where use of alcohol and eating certain meats can provoke attacks. People with gout should discuss this with their physicians.) In rare cases, food allergies can cause attacks of arthritis. There is some evidence that eating oils from cold-water fish can help people with rheumatoid arthritis; however, the bene-fit is small. Of course, it is not wise to be overweight, because that places an extra burden on joints. Most people with chronic arthritis should eat balanced, pleasur-able meals and maintain a normal weight. Ways to do this are discussed in Chapter 13.

It is not surprising that sometimes in the struggle against arthritis, an individual becomes depressed. It is important to *recognize the depression* and to seek advice from health professionals. There are many ways to combat depression; the impor-tant thing is to know it is present and take steps to control it.

Most people with chronic arthritis are able to lead productive and satisfying, independent lives. The most important step in achieving this is to take an active part in managing your own arthritis. All of the components of management men-tioned here either are the responsibility of the individual or are best done with the individual's participation. The rest of this book is devoted to making your partici-pation most effective.

Community Resource Detective's Kit

Arthritis Information

Arthritis Foundation, 1314 Spring Street NW, Atlanta, GA 30309, (800) 283-7800 for local chapter.
http://www.arthritis.org

Arthritis Today Magazine—for subscription contact the Arthritis Foundation or call (800) 933-0032.

National Arthritis and Musculoskeletal and Skin Diseases Information Clearinghouse (NAMISIC), P. O. Box AMS, 9000 Rockville Pike, Bethesda, MD 20892, (301) 495-4484.
http://www.nih.gov/niams/healthinfo/(info)

•••

Suggested Further Reading

Arthritis Foundation staff. *Living Better with Fibromyalgia.* Atlanta, Ga.: Arthritis Foundation, 1996.

Backstrom, Gayle. *The Relief Handbook for Fibromyalgia and Chronic Muscle Pain: When Muscle Pain Won't Go Away.* Dallas: Taylor Publishing, 1995.

Davidson, Paul. *Are You Sure It's Arthritis? A Guide to Soft-Tissue Rheumatism.* New American Library, 1987.

Fries, James F. *Arthritis: A Comprehensive Guide to Understanding Your Arthritis,* 5th ed. Reading, Mass.: Perseus, 2000.

Fries, James F. *Arthritis: A Take Care of Yourself Health Guide.* Reading, Mass.: Addison-Wesley, 1995.

Horstman, Judith. *The Arthritis Foundation's Guide to Alternative Therapies.* Atlanta, Ga.: Arthritis Foundation, 1999.

Lorig, Kate, and James Fries. *The Arthritis Helpbook*, 5th ed. Reading, Mass.: Perseus, 2000.

Sayce, Valerie, and Ian Fraser. *Exercise Beats Arthritis: An Easy-to-Follow Program of Exercise,* 3rd ed. Palo Also, Calif.: Bull Publishing, 1998.

CHAPTER
18

Understanding Diabetes

WHILE DIABETES IS A SERIOUS DISEASE, YOU CAN LIVE A LONG AND healthy life and prevent complications. Living well with diabetes requires both good medical care and effective self-management. Although there is much that health care providers can do, you must take responsibility for learning about diabetes and managing the daily decisions and actions necessary to deal with the disease. Before looking at all the options for self-managment, however, let's talk about diabetes and its causes.

What Is Diabetes?

Diabetes is essentially a disease that makes it difficult for the body to turn food into fuel. To understand diabetes, it is helpful to know a little about the digestion process, the function of the pancreas and insulin in the body, and how these relate to diabetes. (See Figure 18.1.)

Some of the food we eat (carbohydrates and sugars) is broken down in the digestion process into a simple sugar called glucose. The glucose is absorbed into the bloodstream from your stomach, which makes your blood glucose (also known as blood sugar) levels rise. In order for the cells of your body to use the glucose as fuel, it needs the help of insulin. Insulin is a hormone produced by the pancreas, a small gland located below and behind your stomach. Insulin acts as a bridge that helps the blood glucose get from the bloodstream into the cells. Once inside the cells, the glucose is burned to give your body energy.

Glucose in the body can be compared to the gasoline in a car; they are both a fuel and a source of energy. Gasoline alone, however, is not enough to make the car move. We also need a key to start the motor, which allows the gasoline to be

Figure 18.1 *The Digestion Process*

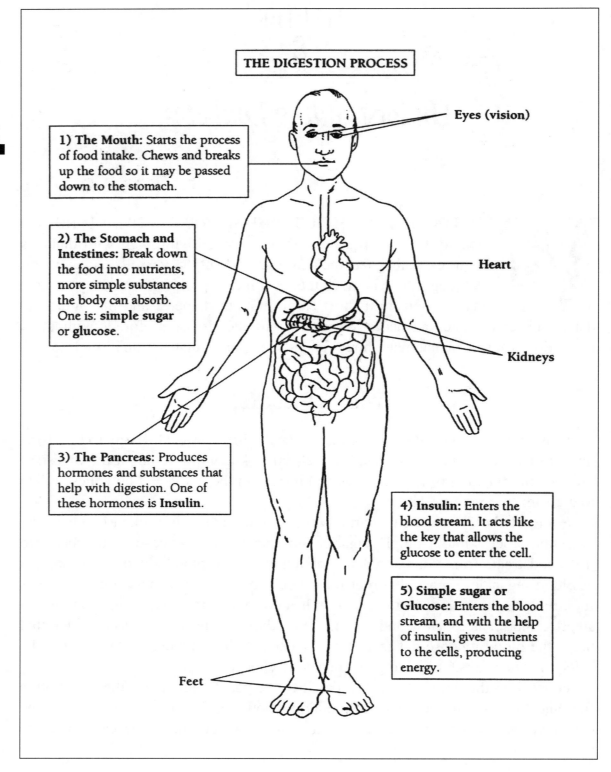

THE DIGESTION PROCESS

Eyes (vision)

1) The Mouth: Starts the process of food intake. Chews and breaks up the food so it may be passed down to the stomach.

2) The Stomach and Intestines: Break down the food into nutrients, more simple substances the body can absorb. One is: **simple sugar** or **glucose**.

Heart

Kidneys

3) The Pancreas: Produces hormones and substances that help with digestion. One of these hormones is **Insulin**.

4) Insulin: Enters the blood stream. It acts like the key that allows the glucose to enter the cell.

5) Simple sugar or Glucose: Enters the blood stream, and with the help of insulin, gives nutrients to the cells, producing energy.

Feet

converted into energy. Like the car, our bodies also need a key that enables us to use glucose as energy. Insulin is this key; it carries the glucose from the bloodstream into the cells where it produces energy for the body.

In diabetes, insulin is not able to carry out this function, because either the pancreas does not produce enough insulin or the insulin that is produced cannot be used efficiently by the body. As a result, glucose rises to high levels in the blood. When the kidneys filter the blood, excess glucose spills out in the urine. This causes one of the symptoms of diabetes, which is frequent urination and large amounts of sugar in the urine. This is how diabetes got its name, *diabetes mellitus.* The Greek word *diabetes* means "to pass through," and the Latin word *mellitus* means "sugar" or "honey."

There are different types of diabetes. Table 18.1 provides a comparison of the two most common types, Type 1 and Type 2 diabetes. There is one thing common for all types of diabetes: The body does not produce enough insulin, or it cannot use the insulin that is produced.

As is the case for so many chronic diseases, the exact cause of diabetes is not known. Type 1 diabetes, also known as *insulin-dependent diabetes,* usually starts in childhood; it is probably an autoimmune disease. This means that for reasons we do not completely understand, the body turns on its immune system to destroy the pancreas' ability to produce insulin. The result is a lack or absence of insulin.

Type 2 diabetes, often referred to as *non-insulin-dependent diabetes,* or *adult-onset diabetes mellitus,* usually starts in adulthood after age 40. Although there is no single cause for Type 2 diabetes, its onset appears to be related to a series of factors. It is more common among people who are overweight, where the excess fat does not allow the body to use the insulin well. In other words, insulin is produced, but the body is resistant to it. Insulin resistance means that the body is not very effective in moving the glucose from the blood into the cells of the body. Therefore, the glucose builds up in the blood because the body cannot use it.

Type 2 diabetes does not seem to be an autoimmune disease. Rather, it tends to run in families and its onset may occur as a result of other factors such as being overweight, stress, eating, and other lifestyle habits or some other illness.

The important difference between the two types of diabetes is that Type 1 requires the daily use of insulin, whereas the majority of people with Type 2 do not need insulin to control the disease. Despite this difference, however, there are some similarities in the symptons that can appear in both types of diabetes. These include fatigue, increased appetite, blurry vision, frequent urination, excessive thirst, changes in mood, infections, and unexplained weight loss.

Table 18.1 *Overview of Type I and Type II Diabetes*

Characteristics	Type 1 Diabetes (insulin dependent)	Type 2 Diabetes (may or may not need insulin and may need oral medications)
Age	Usually begins before age 20, but can occur in adults	Usually begins after age 40, but can occur earlier
Insulin	Little or no insulin is produced by the pancreas	The pancreas produces insulin, but it may not be enough or it cannot be used by the body
Onset	Sudden	Slow
Sex	Males and females equally affected	More females are affected
Heredity	Some hereditary tendency	Strong hereditary tendency
Weight	Majority experience weight loss and are thin	Majority are overweight
Ketones	Ketones found in the urine	Usually there are no ketones in the urine
Treatment	Insulin, diet, exercise, self-management	Diet, exercise, self-management, and when necessary, oral medication and/or insulin

Self-Management

No matter what kind of diabetes you have, there are two major self-management tasks to keep in mind. The first is to maintain a safe blood glucose level. This means balancing all the treatment methods, which include healthy eating, exercise, managing stress and emotions, and medication. The second task is to detect early any problems caused by diabetes. Of course, these two are very closely linked because high blood glucose levels cause many of these problems. Let's examine these management tasks in more detail.

275

Maintaining a Safe Blood Glucose Level

We know that the body gets nutrients and glucose through the digestive process. The blood carries this glucose to the body's cells where it is converted into energy. Therefore, it is important to have a certain amount of glucose in your blood all the time, for your body to use for energy throughout the day. The goal of diabetes management is to maintain a blood glucose level appropriate for your condition. Normal blood glucose levels fall within the range of 80–120 mg/dL; however, not all people with diabetes can have a "normal" level. Discuss with your doctor what blood glucose level you should try to maintain. The problems occur when the blood glucose level is either too high, called *hyperglycemia,* or too low, *hypoglycemia.* It is helpful to understand the causes and symptoms of high and low blood glucose (see Tables 18.2 and 18.3) as well as what to do if your blood glucose level is too high or low (see below).

Your job as a self-manager is to keep your blood sugar at an appropriate level, not too high or too low. This is achieved by maintaining a balance through your eating plan, exercise, and, when necessary, the use of medicines. In addition, strong emotions and illness can also affect blood glucose levels; therefore, knowing how to manage these effectively can help in controlling your diabetes.

Managing a Healthy Eating Plan

The way you eat makes a big difference in controlling your diabetes. However, for many people with diabetes, going on "diets" or making changes in eating habits can seem overwhelming at first. Remember, small changes in your eating can make important differences in your blood glucose levels and how you feel. Also, healthy eating can still be tasty, satisfying, and fun.

You do not have to go hungry or deprive yourself of the foods you like best, nor do you have to buy "special" food. An eating plan that is good for diabetes is also a healthier diet for all family members. Rather, you need to be careful only about the quantity and quality of the foods you eat so that each meal is nutritionally balanced.

Table 18.2 *Causes of Hyperglycemia and Hypoglycemia*

Hyperglycemia (too high blood glucose level)	Hypoglycemia (too low blood glucose level)
Too little or poorly timed oral medication	Too much or poorly timed insulin or diabetes medications/ pills
Too much food, especially sweet foods or drinks, or foods high in carbohydrates	Not eating regularly or eating less than usual
Poorly timed or irregular meals	Eating at irregular hours, missing or skipping meals
Less exercise or physical activity than usual Emotional stress	More exercise or physical activity than usual or poorly timed exercise Emotional stress
Medication is bad (it was frozen, got too hot, or is too old)	Drinking alcohol on an empty stomach
Illness such as fever, colds or flu, or surgery	

To do this, however, you may need to make changes in some of your eating habits. For example, you may need to eat more of some foods and less of others, eat a greater variety of foods, establish a regular schedule for your meals, and/or eat the same quantity or portions at each meal.

All foods contain nutrients that provide the body with energy. For people with diabetes, there are three types of nutrients that are important to consider when watching the way you eat: carbohydrates, proteins, and fats. Carbohydrates (simple and complex) cause blood glucose levels to rise more rapidly than do proteins or fats. For this reason, it is important to watch the total amount of carbohydrates you eat at each meal. The goal is to choose vegetables, fruits, grains, and pasta. These types of carbohydrates provide good nutrients, energy, and fiber but fewer calories and less fat. Try to limit carbohydrates with simple sugars such as candy,

Table 18.3 *Symptoms of Hyperglycemia and Hypoglycemia*

Hyperglycemia	Hypoglycemia
Usually, slow onset (days or months)	Usually, sudden onset (hours or minutes)
Unusual, excessive thirst	Cold, clammy skin or sweating
Frequent urination	Hard, fast heartbeat
Fatigue, extreme tiredness	Hunger
Blurry vision	Numbness or tingling (in fingers and toes)
Frequent or persistent infections	Confusion, nervousness, or irritability
Unexplained weight loss	Slurred speech
Nausea and vomiting	Headache
Deep, rapid breathing	Convulsions, night sweats
Fruity-smelling breath	Restless sleep
High level of ketones in the urine	Unconsciousness

cakes, cookies, sodas, and ice cream, which not only rapidly raise your blood glucose but also add fat and calories. This doesn't mean you can never have a slice of birthday cake again. Remember, moderation is the key to successful management of blood glucose.

Proteins are needed to repair muscle tissues, bones, and skin; they also supply energy for the body in the absence of carbohydrates. Generally, proteins are found in animal products like meat, fish, milk, and so on, as well as in vegetables and grain products. As animal proteins tend to be high in fat, try to choose low-fat sources of protein. Fats are also used by the body for energy and help absorb certain vitamins. They are necessary for the body but, if consumed in excess, can lead to weight gain and affect the heart and other organs, complicating your diabetes even more. Choose low-fat or nonfat foods often. You will find more detailed information about nutrition and guidelines for healthy eating in Chapter 13.

The eating plan for a person with diabetes is similar to that recommended for everyone: one that encourages you to eat a variety of foods. This has many advantages. Besides helping you to maintain an appropriate blood sugar level, it also helps you maintain a healthy weight, as well as reduce your blood pressure and cholesterol.

The person with diabetes, however, needs to be more careful than other people when it comes to how much and when to eat. The type, amount, and timing of meals all affect your blood sugar level. Watch the size of the portions of food you eat. Most people would benefit from smaller portions. It is generally better to eat smaller meals every 4–5 hours during the day, and be sure not to skip breakfast. To keep your blood sugar within your appropriate range, it is especially important to balance when you eat with the time you exercise and/or take medication.

To learn more about managing your eating plan, we recommend that you spend some time with a certified diabetes educator. This is a person who has been specially trained to teach diabetes management and is certified by the American Association of Diabetes Educators. A nutritionist or dietician can also help you tailor your eating plan to fit with your lifestyle. Some additional resources are listed at the end of this chapter.

Exercise

Regular physical activity is one of the best things you can do to control diabetes and improve health. Exercise provides all the benefits for the person with diabetes that it does for everyone else. It keeps the joints flexible, strengthens the heart, lungs, and blood vessels to help prevent heart problems, reduces stress, and helps many people deal with sad or unhappy feelings. And remember, no one is too old to start some gentle physical activity.

Since many people with diabetes are also overweight, exercise provides the added benefits of burning calories and lowering your blood sugar level. This, in turn, helps you to lose weight and/or maintain an appropriate weight. Exercise helps with weight control in three ways. First, we burn calories or energy while we are exercising. Second, exercise helps build and maintain muscle. Therefore, a steady supply of energy in the form of glucose needs to be supplied because the muscles are burning calories (using energy) 24 hours a day. This helps manage weight. Third, sustained aerobic exercise, which is exercise that raises your heart rate, makes you breathe harder or perspire and also increases the rate at which the body burns calories. For example, after 30 minutes, the body will start to burn calories from fat to obtain the energy it needs to function; therefore, you are burning calories through an increase in your metabolism, as well as through exercise. When you stop exercising, your metabolism does not return immediately to normal. It remains somewhat elevated for up to 6 hours after. Exercise changes the metabolism in the muscles and helps normalize blood glucose levels. Thus, you continue burning calories at an increased rate long after you finish exercising, helping your body use the glucose in the blood as energy. Strenuous exercise may lower blood glucose for up to 36 hours. The good news is that all it takes to increase your metabolism is 20–30 minutes of regular aerobic exercise. Thus, everyone with diabetes should have a goal of some type of aerobic activity, such as walking, bicycling, swimming, or dancing, for 30 minutes at least four times a week. However, it's fine to build up slowly. Even 5 minutes of gentle physical activity can make a big difference and brings you closer to your goal.

Exercise is an important part of your self-management program because it helps to lower your blood sugar. However, sometimes it can lower your blood sugar too much, which can cause hypoglycemia and other problems. Therefore, it is important to find the best time during the day to exercise and to know how to treat hypoglycemia should it occur. Generally, the best time to exercise is when your blood sugar tends to be the highest, which is usually 1–2 hours after a meal. If you are not sure, discuss this with your doctor or diabetes educator. They can also tell you what steps you should take to treat hypoglycemia. These are mentioned on page 286 in this chapter.

For more information on how to develop and maintain an exercise program, see Chapter 6. Also, be sure to read page 139 for some special advice on exercise for people with diabetes.

Stress and Emotions

After learning that you have diabetes, you may be feeling angry, scared, or depressed. These feelings are normal, understandable, and manageable. For people with diabetes, stress and emotions such as anger, fear, frustration, and depression can affect blood sugar levels. For this reason, it is important to learn effective ways to deal with these feelings. Don't try to hide or suppress your emotions; these are a normal part of life and some of the work you will have to deal with in managing your condition. To help you understand the impact of these feelings on your illness and identify some ways to manage them, read Chapters 4, 5, and 10.

Other Illnesses

When a person with diabetes is sick with an infection, a cold, or the flu, the blood sugar tends to go up, and food and medicines can have different effects during those days. For this reason, it is especially important to have a plan for sick days and know what to do and when to seek additional help. Therefore, be sure you have the following on hand to help you manage your sick days:

- A family member or friend who is ready and able to help you when needed. This person should also know what to do to help you and when to call the doctor or when to take you to the emergency room, if needed.
- Have plenty of both sweetened and unsweetened or sugarless liquids on hand.
- Have a thermometer at home and learn how to use it.
- Have your emergency medical information on hand (including doctor's number, list of medications and dosages, and so on).

Be sure to ask your doctor or nurse under what circumstances they want you to call them. The accompanying box provides some general guidelines for when to call the doctor if your sick day self-care steps are not working for you.

Insulin Injection

Insulin is used to treat everyone with Type 1 diabetes and for some people with Type 2 diabetes. It is used to replace the insulin that is not produced and/or adequately utilized by the body. Insulin is taken by injection. There are three types of insulin, classified according to how long they work to lower blood glucose. Table 18.4 provides a brief overview of these types of insulin. It is important that you know the type of insulin you are taking, the company that makes it, the dose (number of units you are taking), and that the insulin you are taking has not passed its expiration date. If you feel that you could benefit from learning more about the use of insulin, talk with your doctor or diabetes educator. You will also find a list of resources at the end of this chapter.

Diabetes Medications/Pills

Most people with Type 2 diabetes do not take insulin. They can control their diabetes with a healthy eating plan and exercise and, sometimes, with diabetes medications in pill form. Many people with Type 2 diabetes can avoid taking insulin or other diabetes medications by controlling their weight. Sometimes, one

What to Do When You Are Sick

- Test your blood glucose more frequently. If possible, monitor it every 4 hours and write down the results. This will help you make decisions about your food, medicines, and when to call the doctor.

- Drink ½ cup of fluids every hour, according to your blood sugar level. If you have *high* blood sugar, drink nonsugary liquid; if you have *low* blood sugar, drink ½ cup of sugar liquid for a total of 1 cup before testing blood again.

- Keep taking your medication unless you are vomiting or have diarrhea, in which case, call your doctor.

- Tell a family member or friend how you're feeling so that they are aware of your condition and can help you. Ask them to check on you 3 to 4 times a day.

- Call the doctor if any of the following occurs:
  - The above self-care steps do not help you improve within 24–48 hours.
  - Your blood sugar is above 300 for more than 2 days.
  - Your temperature is above 101°F (38.3°C) or above 100°F (37.8°C) for 2 days.
  - You have been vomiting or have had diarrhea for more than 1 day.
  - You are not able to drink liquids or food for more than 8 hours.
  - If you have Type 1 diabetes, call the doctor if your glucose is 240 mg/dL or over for 2 days or your blood glucose is much higher than usual for you.
  - Your blood glucose is less than 60 twice in one day.
  - You have "moderate" or "large" ketones in your urine for more than 8 hours.
  - You are not feeling well and are unsure of what you should do to care for yourself.

When you do call your doctor or nurse, be prepared with the following information: the type of diabetes you have, your blood sugar level (if you know it), your temperature, if you have ketones in your urine, symptoms, the medications you are taking, and what you have done to treat your symptoms.

Table 18.4 *Types of Insulin*

Type	Onset of Action	Maximum Effect	Duration
Short acting (regular)	½–1 hour	2–5 hours	6–8 hours
Intermediate acting (NPH or lente)	1–2 hours	6–12 hours	18–24 hours
Long acting (ultralente)	4–8 hours	12–18 hours	24–28 hours
Mixed rapid and intermediate acting	½ hour	4–12 hours	18–24 hours

Remember that not all brands (even of the same type) act exactly the same. These are general guidelines. To find out specific information about your insulin, ask your doctor or pharmacist.

needs to lose only 10–15 pounds (4–6 kg) to normalize blood glucose. Table 18.5 lists the most common medications used for non-insulin diabetes.

Some people take pills to help lower their blood glucose levels. Know what kinds of medications you take and how often to take them. It is very helpful to carry a card in your wallet listing your medications and dosages. The diabetes medications may work to increase insulin secretion, slow absorption of carbohydrates from the stomach, decrease glucose production in the liver, and/or increase the sensitivity of body cells to use insulin. Know when to take your medications and don't skip a dose. Most of these drugs are taken once or twice a day, usually right before meals. The medications do *not* take the place of healthy eating and regular physical activity. Check with your doctor before stopping or changing your medicines even if you don't feel well. Always keep your medications with you (not in your luggage) when traveling.

Other medications can sometimes interact with diabetes pills. Therefore, it is important that your doctor and pharmacist know all the medications you are taking, including prescription and nonprescription.

Table 18.5 *Medications Used for Non-Insulin-Dependent Diabetes*

Name of Medication	How It Works
Sulfonylureas: tolazamide (Tolinase), tolbutamide, (Orinase), glipizide (Glucotrol), glyburide, (DiaBeta, Micronase), chlorpropamide (Diabinese)	Increased insulin secretion
Alpha-glucosidase inhibitors: acrabose (Precose)	Slows digestion and absorption of carbohydrates
Biguanides: Metformin (Glucophage)	Decreases glucose production in liver
Thiazolidenediones: troglitazone (Rezulin)	Increases use of insulin in muscle cells, decreases insulin resistance

In general, it is a good idea to avoid alcohol. For the person with diabetes, alcohol can cause a sudden and drastic drop in blood glucose, and it adds calories that can lead to weight gain. When alcohol is taken with oral diabetes medications, especially Diabinese, it can sometimes cause problems such as flushing, tingling, and light-headedness. Thus, be careful and limit your consumption of alcohol. If you do drink, make sure you have some food with it to avoid a low blood sugar reaction that can happen if you have alcohol on an empty stomach.

Timing and Balance

Now that we have talked about food, exercise, emotions, illnesses, and medications, we must mention timing and balance. All of these factors are related and interact in helping to maintain the blood glucose level. For example, increased exercise may lower blood glucose, and this may allow you to increase the amount you eat or reduce (under the guidance of your doctor) the dosage of your diabetes medication. To understand and monitor the effects of food, exercise, illnesses, and medications, it is helpful to learn how to test your blood sugar at home (see below).

As mentioned earlier, diabetes management depends on the ability to balance these different areas. This is something you must learn to do, and it can be achieved by making changes in your habits and incorporating them into your daily life. To get more guidance with this, talk to your doctor or diabetes educator. Also, the resources at the end of this chapter may be helpful.

Home Blood Glucose Monitoring

284

So far we have discussed the basic things you can do to manage your diabetes. Another important area is learning to monitor your blood glucose level. As we said at the beginning, keeping your blood glucose level under control is a balancing act. Of course there are the tests that your doctor can do to monitor your condition, including the blood glucose tests (fasting or nonfasting) and the hemoglobin A1C. However, the most important tests are the ones you do at home on a daily basis.

Monitoring your blood glucose helps you know if the strategies you are using to control your diabetes are working. Only through monitoring and recording the results can you judge the success of your program and make appropriate adjustments. It is important to monitor your blood glucose regularly. How often to test is generally determined by how unstable your blood glucose levels are, what medications you are taking, and how you feel. You can work out an appropriate plan with your doctor and diabetes educator. Below we discuss the different ways that people with diabetes monitor ther blood glucose level, as well as the advantages and disadvantages of each method.

Observing Symptoms

While it is important to recognize and know how you feel when your blood glucose is very low or high, this is not the best method for controlling your diabetes for two reasons. First, many people do not even experience symptoms until their blood sugar is already very high or low. This makes it very difficult to stay within their appropriate blood glucose range. Second, many of the symptoms that someone might experience can be similar for both conditions: high and low blood sugar. Without knowing what the actual blood glucose level is, it is difficult to determine what steps to take to treat it.

Urine Testing

In the past, the method many people used to see if there was sugar in the blood was the urine test. When there gets to be a certain high level of sugar in the blood, it is eliminated in the urine. Therefore, you could test the urine to see if this occurred. Usually this test is done in the morning before eating, using a special strip that is dipped into the urine. If the strip changes color, this means that the level of blood sugar is too high. Unfortunately, this method tells you only when the blood sugar level is too high, not when it may be too low. Urine testing cannot help you determine how specific activities, such as eating, exercise, stressful events, medications, and so on, affect your blood sugar levels during the day and over time. Also, certain medications can affect the accuracy of the urine test results.

Home Blood Glucose Testing

The main method of self-monitoring is testing your blood. This is a simple test that can be done at home or anywhere. To do the test, you need a small device called a *blood* glucose monitor or meter and test strips. There are several different types of meters, but all require that you prick the tip of your finger with a sterile needle to get a drop of blood. This droplet is then placed on a strip and put into the meter. Within seconds, the meter gives a reading of your blood glucose level. This test helps you keep track of how well you are balancing your eating, exercise, and medications during the day and over time. For this reason, this is the most efficient method for helping you control your blood sugar and make the necessary adjustments in your self-management program.

What Do I Do If . . . ?

Blood glucose levels can be too low (hypoglycemia) or too high (hyperglycemia). In some cases, blood sugar can fluctuate widely; this usually happens when there is not an appropriate balance among the factors we discussed earlier: food, exercise, and medication (refer to Table 18.2, on page 276, for the different possible causes).

Hypoglycemia

When your blood glucose is too low (less than 60 mg/dL), you may experience symptoms such as dizziness, cold sweats, shakiness, and so on (see Table 18.3, page 277), which if not treated immediately can lead to an emergency situation. Therefore, it is important to raise your blood sugar quickly (see the box "Steps for Treating Low Blood Sugar" on the next page).

For the person with diabetes, it is important to always carry one of these "remedy" or sugary foods with you and to know when to get medical help for treating low blood sugar. Therefore, we recommend you call the doctor or nurse for help if

- you have repeated episodes of low blood sugar (more than three) within a week,

- your blood sugar is repeatedly lower than usual without cause, or

- you need help from another person when your blood sugar is low.

Also, we recommend that a person with diabetes wear an emergency bracelet and/or carry an emergency card in her or his wallet. The emergency card should also have information about medication, doctor, and emergency contact person's name and number. This will help people know what to do and who to contact in case of emergency.

Steps for Treating Low Blood Sugar

1. *Check your blood sugar immediately* if possible to see how low it is.

2. *Eat a "remedy" or sugary food* (for example, 5–7 Lifesavers, 3–4 glucose tablets, 3 packets of sugar, 1 handful of raisins, a small tube of cake icing, or 1 tablespoon of honey).

3. *Wait 15 minutes, note your symptoms, and check your blood sugar again* (if possible).

4. *If, after 15 minutes, the symptoms are not better or there is no change in your blood sugar level, repeat steps 2 and 3* (eat another remedy food and wait 15 minutes).

5. *If your symptoms are not better after repeating these steps a few times, call the doctor or nurse.* Do not wait—it is important to get medical help.

6. *If your symptoms are better and your next meal is more than 1 hour away, eat a snack* (for example, ½ sandwich, low-fat cheese, crackers, or a cup of milk).

Hyperglycemia

When your blood glucose gets too high (more than 240 mg/dL), this is considered hyperglycemia. This usually occurs gradually and sometimes without symptoms. If there are symptoms, they can include extreme thirst, frequent urination, fatigue, blurry vision, and so on (see Table 18.3, page 277). Like hypoglycemia, hyperglycemia can occur when your diet, exercise, and/or medications are out of balance. It can be caused by eating too much food, especially eating sweets and fatty foods, lack of exercise, and/or not enough medication (see Table 18.2, page 276). Fortunately, hyperglycemia can be monitored with daily blood testing. If you begin to notice a pattern in which your blood sugar is rising, you may want to watch carefully how much and what you are eating, increase your exercise, and talk to your doctor or nurse about possible changes in your medication.

If you have diabetes and get another illness (for example, a cold), you should also monitor you blood glucose carefully and follow the recommendations for what to do when you are sick, on page 281.

Preventing the Complications of Diabetes

Unfortunately, poor diabetes control can lead to other complications. These complications include damage to the cardiovascular system or heart disease, nerve damage (neuropathy, which causes burning, tingling, or numbness in the hands and feet), liver and kidney damage, vision problems, bladder infections, and gum disease. Because diabetes can silently progress and damage other organs of the body, it is important to practice the following measures to prevent these more serious complications:

- Maintain your blood sugar within an acceptable range (80–120 mg/dL or as recommended by your doctor).
- Do home blood glucose testing regularly and keep a written record.
- Have regular checkups with your doctor including:
  - Remind your doctor to check your feet at each visit. (Refer to page 290 for other tips about foot care.)
  - Have blood glucose/HgA1C* levels checked several times a year.**
  - Have your eyes (including retina at the back of your eyeball) examined every 1 to 2 years** and report any changes in vision to your doctor.

---

* The hemoglobin A1C (HA1C) or glycosylated hemoglobin is a blood test that measures the average control of blood glucose over a several-month period. Therefore, it has an advantage over a single blood glucose measurement that may be high or low at that specific time due to diet, exercise, medications, illness, or whatever.
** Or as recommended by your doctor.

- Check your blood pressure yearly.**
- Have your cholesterol and lipids checked yearly.**
- Have your kidney function checked yearly.**

- Have a yearly influenza vaccine and a once-per-lifetime pneumoccal pneumonia vaccine.

- At every visit, remind the doctor and nurse that you have diabetes.

- Practice proper foot care at home (see the suggestions on page 290).

- Protect your skin. Don't get sunburned, and keep your skin clean.

- Clean and floss your teeth daily.

- Have regular checkups with the dentist.

- Stop smoking and/or avoid being around smoke.

- Set personal goals to control your diabetes and review/revise them regularly.

- Attend a diabetes education program to learn more about your condition.

Heart Disease

Heart disease occurs because there is a tendency for the walls of the blood vessels to harden more quickly when blood sugar levels are elevated. This leads to poor circulation and obstruction in the arteries, which is the principal problem in heart disease and can cause a heart attack. The hardening of the arteries and the risk of heart disease can be reduced, however, when a near-normal level of blood glucose is maintained. This can be achieved by paying careful attention to a low-fat diet and a regular aerobic exercise routine.

Infection

Infections of the skin, bladder, kidneys, vagina, or gums occur because the cells of the immune system are not as effective at killing the bacteria or viruses that enter the body when blood sugar levels are high. Also, if your blood sugar is high, there is more likely to be more sugar in your urine, which stimulates the growth of microorganisms that can cause infections. If your diabetes is poorly controlled, your body's capacity to defend itself against infection is diminished. For this reason, it is important to control your blood glucose levels and to treat any injury or infection immediately. It is also important to take good care of your skin, keeping it clean and dry and using a moisturizer to keep it from drying out. This is especially true and necessary when taking care of your feet.

Foot Problems

People with diabetes have several reasons for being concerned about their feet. First, there is the problem of infection due to the decrease in blood circulation to the legs and feet. This is why little cuts and sores do not heal well and become infected. Next, since the feet are a long way from the heart, sometimes they do not get all the blood they need. This is especially true if there is some narrowing of the blood vessels. When the feet do not get enough blood, the tissue not only has too much sugar, it does not have enough oxygen. Oxygen is needed to prevent tissue damage and to help the healing process.

When people also have nerve damage (neuropathy) from diabetes, they often have numbness in the feet. This can cause the feet to be less sensitive to heat, cold, and pain. Thus, when any injury occurs, you may not be able to feel it until the damage is quite severe. For this reason, it is important to practice good foot care regularly, following the suggestions on page 290. Also, if you do have problems with your feet, you may want to consult with a foot specialist (podiatrist).

Vision Problems

Blurred vision is very common with high blood sugar levels but can also occur with low blood sugar. The blurring goes away, however, when the blood glucose is brought under control. Of more concern is a condition called *diabetic retinopathy,* in which the small blood vessels of the eye become hard and break, causing damage to the retina (the light-sensitive membrane located in the back of the eye). This damage can cause vision problems and sometimes blindness. The condition can often be controlled if caught early.

With good control of the blood glucose level, the risk of serious eye problems can be reduced. Therefore, it is very important that every person with diabetes have a retinal eye examination with an eye doctor (ophthalmologist) yearly or as recommended by your doctor. When you go for this exam, be sure to tell the doctor that you have diabetes and that you especially want him or her to check for diabetic retinopathy. This retinal exam is different from a test by an optometrist, who checks your vision to see if you need glasses or corrective lenses.

Nerve Damage

Nerve damage, or neuropathy, is very common in people with diabetes. The symptoms range from burning pain and numbness in the feet, legs, or hands to dizziness upon standing. A person with neuropathy may also have sexual problems such as impotence or vaginal dryness. Everything that is controlled by the nerves can be affected one way or another by diabetes. Neuropathy can be prevented

For Proper Foot Care, Remember to . . .

- *Check your feet every day.* You or someone else should look between the toes and on the tops and bottoms of the feet for cuts or sores (e.g., corns, calluses, or blisters), ingrown toenails, extreme dryness, bruises, redness, swelling, or pus.

- *Wash your feet every day.* Use mild soap and warm water. Be sure to test the water's temperature with your elbow first. DO NOT SOAK your feet.

- *Dry your feet well between the toes.*

- *Cut your toenails straight across.* Do not cut the back corners of the nail. If you can't safely trim your toenails, ask a family member to do it or get professional help. Also, do not clean under your toenails or remove skin with sharp objects.

- *Rub a mild lotion on your feet before bed if the skin is dry* (except between the toes).

- *Wear comfortable shoes and socks* (never go barefoot except when bathing or in bed). Your shoes should support, protect, and cover your feet. If your feet sweat, use powder. Check inside your shoes before putting them on, and break in new shoes gradually. Also, avoid socks with tight, elastic tops.

- *Have your doctor check your feet.* When you go to the doctor, take off your shoes and socks so that your feet can be easily examined.

or controlled by keeping your blood sugar level within your normal range, so discuss any symptoms with your doctor.

Your Role Is Important

Please note that most of the problems mentioned above can be treated and prevented, but you have an important role in doing so. First, maintain your blood glucose level within your normal range. This will help prevent or reduce complications; if problems occur, good blood glucose control can prevent them from

Community Resource Detective's Kit

Diabetes Resources

American Diabetes Association (ADA)
1660 Duke Street,
P.O. Box 25757, Alexandria, VA 22313
http://www.diabetes.org

The ADA publishes a magazine bimonthly called Diabetes Forecast. *It is filled with practical tips on diabetes care and relates personal experiences of people with diabetes.*

International Diabetes Center
4959 Excelsior Boulevard
Minneapolis, MN 55416
http://www.Idcdiabetes.org

The center offers a variety of inexpensive pamphlets, booklets, and slide sets dealing with various facets of diabetes care.

Joslin Diabetes Foundation, Inc.
One Joslin Place
Boston, MA 02215
http://www.joslin.harvard.edu/

This world-famous facility has separate divisions for research, education, and youth. Their efforts involve all facets of diabetes management and research. It is one of eight Diabetes Research and Training Centers designated by the National Institute of Health.

National Diabetes Information Clearinghouse
7910 Woodmont Avenue, Suite 1811
Bethesda, MD 10014
http://www.aoa.dhhs.gov/aoa/dir/153.html

This organization publishes a list of nutrition information related to diabetes management.

becoming worse. Second, be aware of your body and symptoms. If you detect something early, such as an infection or eye problems, it will be easier to treat.

As with all chronic conditions, diabetes is a disease that can be greatly controlled through good self-management. The path is not always easy, but it can be beneficial to your overall health when successfully followed.

To become a good diabetes self-manager, there is much more to learn than what is discussed in this chapter. Therefore, be sure to talk to your doctor or diabetes educator about your questions, problems, and/or concerns. Try to find other information and resources in your community to help you become the best of self-managers. Some resources are listed at the end of this chapter that may help you start.

•••

Suggested Further Reading

Cryer, Philip E. *American Diabetes Association Complete Guide to Diabetes: The Ultimate Home Diabetes Reference.* New York: Bantam Books, 1992.

Joslin, Elliot P., C. Ronald Kahn, and Gordon C. Weir. *Joslin's Diabetes Mellitus.* Philadelphia: Lea and Febiger, 1994.

Lowe, Ernest, and Gary Arsham. *Diabetes: A Guide to Living Well.* Wayzuta, Minn.: Diabetes Center, Inc., 1989.

Milchovich, Sue, and Barbara Dunn-Long. *Diabetes Mellitus, A Practical Handbook,* 7th ed. Palo, Alto, Calif.: Bull Publishing, 1999.

Raymond, Mike. *The Human Side of Diabetes.* Chicago: Noble Press, 1992.

Schade, David S., Patrick J. Boyle, and Mark R. Burge. *101 Tips for Staying Healthy with Diabetes and Avoiding Complications: A Project of the American Diabetes Association.* American Diabetes Association, 1996.

Weiler, Cheryl, Judy Ostrom Jones, Priscilla Hollander, and Marion Franz. *Learning to Live Well with Diabetes.* New York: John Wiley and Sons, 1991.

CHAPTER 19

Planning for the Future: Fears and Reality

P EOPLE WITH CHRONIC ILLNESSES OFTEN WORRY ABOUT WHAT WILL HAPPEN TO them if their disease becomes really disabling. They fear that at some time in the future they may have problems managing their lives and their illness. One way people can deal with fears of the future is to take control and plan for it. They may never need to put their plans into effect, but there is reassurance in knowing that they will still be in control if the events they fear come to pass. Here are the most common concerns and some suggestions that may be useful.

What If I Can't Take Care of Myself Anymore?

Becoming helpless and dependent is one of the most common fears among people with a potentially disabling health problem. This fear usually has physical as well as financial, social, and emotional components.

Physical Concerns of Day-to-Day Living

As your health condition changes over time, you may need to consider changing your living situation. These changes may involve hiring someone to help you in your home or moving to a living situation where help is provided. The decision about which alternative is best will be related to your needs and how best these can be met.

The first thing you will need to do is carefully *evaluate what you can do for yourself* and what activities of daily living (ADLs) will require some kind of help. ADLs are the everyday things like getting out of bed, bathing, dressing, preparing and eating your meals, cleaning house, shopping, paying bills, and so on. Most people can do all of these, even though they may have to do them slowly, with some modification or with some help from gadgets.

Some people, though, may eventually find one or more of these no longer possible without help from somebody else. For example, you may still be able to fix meals, but your mobility may be impaired to the degree that shopping is no longer possible. Or, if you have problems with fainting or sudden bouts of unconsciousness, you might need to have somebody around at all times. Using the problem-solving steps discussed in Chapter 2, analyze and make a list of what the potential problems might be. Once you have this list, problem-solve the problems one at a time, first making a list of every possible solution you can think of.

Example:

Can't go shopping
- Get daughter to shop for me
- Find a volunteer shopping service
- Shop at a store that delivers
- Ask neighbor to shop for me
- Use the internet
- Get home-delivered meals

Can't be by myself
- Hire an around-the-clock attendant
- Move in with a relative
- Get a "Life-Line" emergency response system
- Move to a board and care home
- Move to a retirement community

When you have listed your problems, and the possible solutions to the problems, select the solution that seems the most workable, acceptable, and least expensive for your needs (step 3 of problem solving).

The selection will depend upon your finances, the family or other resources you can call on, and how well any of the potential solutions will in fact solve your problem. Sometimes, one solution will be the answer for several problems. For instance, if you can't shop, can't be alone, and maybe household chores are reaching the point of a foreseeable need for help, you might consider that a retirement home will solve all of these problems, since it offers meals, regular house cleaning, and transportation for errands and medical appointments.

Even if you are not of "retirement" age, many facilities accept younger people, depending on the facility's particular policies. Most facilities for the "retired" take residents as young as 50, or younger if one of a couple is the minimum age. If you are a young person, the local center for people with disabilities or "independent living center" should be able to direct you to an out-of-home care facility appropriate for you.

Your appraisal of your situation and needs may be aided by sitting down with a trusted friend or relative and discussing your abilities and limitations with him or her. Sometimes another person can spot things we ourselves overlook or would like to ignore. A good self-manager often utilizes other resources, which is step 6 in the problem-solving steps in Chapter 2.

Make changes in your life slowly, incrementally. You don't need to change your whole life around to solve one problem. Remember, too, that you can always change your mind, if you don't burn your bridges behind you. If you think that moving out of your own place to another living arrangement (relatives, care home, etc.) would be the thing to do, don't give up your present home until you are settled in your new home and are sure you want to stay there.

If you think you need help with some activities, hiring help at home is less drastic than moving out and may be enough for quite a while. If you can't be alone, and you live with a family member who is away from home during the day, maybe going to an adult or senior day care center will be enough to keep you safe and comfortable while your family is away. In fact, adult day care centers are ideal places to find new friends and activities geared to your abilities.

A social worker at your local senior center, center for people with disabilities, or hospital social services department can be very helpful in providing information about resources in your community and also in giving you ideas about how to deal with your care needs. There are several kinds of professionals who can be of great help. As previously mentioned, *social workers* are good for helping you decide how to solve financial and living arrangement problems and locating appropriate community resources. Some social workers are also trained in counseling the disabled and/or the elderly in relation to emotional and relationship problems that may be associated with your health problem.

A *licensed occupational therapist* can assess your daily living needs and suggest assistive devices or rearrangements in your environment to make life easier.

An *attorney specializing in elder law* should be on your list for helping you set your financial affairs in order to preserve your assets, to prepare a proper will, and perhaps to execute a durable power of attorney for both health care and financial management. If finances are a concern, ask your local senior center for the names of attorneys who offer free or low-cost services to seniors. Your local Bar Association can also refer you to a list of attorneys who are competent in this area. These attorneys are generally familiar with the laws applying to younger persons with disabilities as well. Even if you are not a "senior," your legal needs are much the same as those of the older person.

Finding In-Home Help

If you find that you cannot manage alone, the first option is usually to hire somebody to help. Most people just need a person called a *home aide* or some similar title. These are people who provide no medically related services needing special licensing, but do help with bathing, dressing, meal preparation, and household chores.

There are a number of ways to find somebody. The easiest, but most expensive, is to hire someone through one of the *home care agencies,* usually listed under "home care" or "home nursing" in the telephone book yellow pages. These are usually (but not always) private, for-profit businesses that supply caregiver staff to individuals at home. The fees charged vary with the skill and license of the caregiver and will include an amount for Social Security, insurance, bonding, and profit for the agency.

The fees are usually about double what you would expect to pay for someone you hire directly. The advantage, if you can afford it, is that the agency assumes all payroll responsibilities, including Social Security and federal and state taxes, and responsibility for the skill and integrity of the attendant, and can replace an ill or no-show attendant right away. The agency pays the staff directly. The client has no involvement with paying the attendant, but pays the agency.

Registered nurses (R.N.) hired this way are very expensive, but it is rare that home care for a chronically ill person requires a registered nurse. Licensed vocational nurses (L.V.N.) cost somewhat less, but are still expensive, and are usually not needed unless there are nursing services required (such as dressing changes, injections, ventilator management, etc.). Certified nursing assistants (C.N.A.) have some basic training in nursing, are much less expensive, and can provide satisfactory care for all but the most critically ill person at home.

Most of these agencies also supply home aides as well as licensed staff. Unless you are bedridden, or require some procedure that must be done by someone with a certain category of license, a home aide most likely will be the most appropriate for your needs.

There are registries that supply pre-screened lists of attendants or caregivers, from which you select the one you wish to hire. The agency will charge a "placement fee," usually equal to one month's pay of the person hired. The agency will assume no liability for the skill or honesty of these people, and it will be necessary to check references and interview carefully, just as you would someone who comes from any other source. This type of resource can be found in the yellow pages under the same listing as "home nursing agencies" or "registries." Some agencies provide both their own staff and registries of staff for you to select from.

Other resources that may provide help at home include senior centers and centers serving the disabled population. They often have listings of people who have called them to say they want work as a home attendant, or who have put a notice up on a bulletin board there. These job seekers are not screened, and need to be interviewed carefully and have references checked before they start on the job.

Many experienced home care attendants use the local newspaper's classified "employment wanted" section to find new jobs. Home attendant jobs tend to be temporary, since one's patient usually progresses to a need for more or sometimes less care than they provide, so the attendant must then look for a new job. Again, one can find a competent helper through the newspaper, but the advice to interview carefully is valid here, too.

Probably the best source of help is word of mouth, from somebody who has employed a person or knows of somebody who has worked for someone he or she knows. Putting the word out through your family and social network may result in a jewel.

Home sharing may be a solution for the person who has space and could offer a home to someone in exchange for help. This works best if the help needed consists mainly of household and garden chores. Some people may be willing to provide personal care, such as help with dressing and bathing and meal preparation. Some communities have agencies or government bureaus that help home-sharers and home-sharees locate each other.

Finding Out-of-Home Care

Retirement Communities

The person who needs very little personal care, but recognizes the need to live in a more protected setting, with security, emergency response services, and so on, and who is older (usually over 50) may wish to consider a retirement community. These may be owned units, rental units, or so-called life care facilities. The life care facility requires a substantial advance payment (called an endowment, accommodation fee, or similar label), plus a monthly charge that covers space, services, and, in some cases, personal and/or nursing care when or if the need for that comes. Other such facilities are subsidized (as of this writing) by the federal government for low-income applicants. The criteria for what constitutes low-income are set by the rules governing the federal subsidy that finances the organization.

There are almost always waiting lists for retirement communities, even before they are built and ready for occupancy. If you think such a place would be right for you, you should get on the waiting list right away. You can always change your mind or decline if you are not ready when a space is offered. To locate a facility in your community, call your senior center or go to the library and consult the directory of the *Association of Homes for the Aged.* Your reference librarian should be able to help you find this publication.

Residential Care Homes

Residential care homes, or board and care homes, are licensed by the state or county social services agency. They provide nonmedical care and supervision for those who cannot live alone. These homes fall into two categories, large and small. The small ones have about six residents, who live in a family-like setting in a neighborhood residence. The large ones have more residents, sometimes hundreds, who live in a boardinghouse or hotel-like setting. They take meals in a central dining room and have individual or shared rooms, with activities in large common rooms.

In either type facility, the services to the residents are the same—all meals, assistance with bathing and dressing as needed, laundry, housekeeping, transportation to medical appointments, supervision and assistance with taking medications. In the larger facilities, there are usually professional activities directors. Residents of the larger facilities usually need to be more independent, since there tends not to be as much personal attention as in the smaller homes.

These homes are licensed in most states for either "elderly" (over 62) or "adult" (under 62). The adult category is further divided into facilities for mentally ill, mentally retarded, or physically disabled.

It is important when considering a residential care home to evaluate the type of residents already living there to make sure you will fit in. For example, some of these facilities may cater to individuals who are mentally confused. If you are mentally clear, you would not find much companionship there. If everybody is hard of hearing, you might have trouble finding somebody to talk to.

Although all homes are by law required to provide wholesome meals, you should make sure the cuisine is to your liking and can meet your dietary needs. If you need a salt-free or diabetic diet, for instance, be sure the operator is willing to prepare your special diet.

The monthly fees for residential care homes vary, depending on whether they are spartan or luxurious. The most spartan facilities cost about the same as the SSI (Supplemental Security Income) benefit and will take SSI beneficiaries, billing the government directly. The more luxurious the home is with respect to furnishings, neighborhood, services, etc., the greater the cost. However, even the nicest of these will probably cost less than full-time, 24-hour, seven-days-a-week at-home care.

298

Skilled Nursing Facilities

Sometimes called "nursing homes" or "convalescent hospitals," the skilled nursing facility provides the most comprehensive care for severely ill or disabled people. Typically, a person who has had a stroke or a hip or knee replacement will be transferred from the acute hospital to a skilled nursing facility for a period of rehabilitation before going home. Recent studies have shown that almost half of all people over 65 will spend some time in a nursing home, many of them only for a short time.

No care situation seems to inspire more fear than the prospect of having to go to a nursing home. "Horror stories" in the news media help to foster anxiety about what awful fate will befall anyone who has the misfortune to have to go there.

Public scrutiny is valuable in helping ensure that standards of care and humane and competent treatment are provided. It must be remembered that nursing homes serve a critical need. When one really needs a nursing home, usually no other care situation will meet this need.

Skilled nursing facilities provide medically related care for people who are no longer able to be in a nonmedical care situation. This means that there may be medications to be administered, either by injection or intravenously, or monitored by professional nursing staff. A nursing-home patient is usually very physically limited, needing to have help getting in and out of bed, eating, bathing, or dealing with bladder and/or bowel control. Skilled nursing facilities can also manage care of feeding tubes, respirators, and other high-tech care equipment.

For those who are partially or temporarily disabled, the skilled nursing facility also provides physical, occupational, and speech therapy, wound care, and other therapies.

Not all nursing homes provide all types of care. Some specialize in rehabilitation and therapies, and others specialize in long-term, custodial care. Some are able to provide high-tech nursing services, others do not.

In selecting a nursing home, you should seek out the help of the *hospital discharge planner or social worker,* or a similar professional from a home care agency or center for seniors or the disabled. There are organizations to monitor local nursing homes. Each nursing home is required by law to post in a prominent place the name and phone number of the "ombudsman," a person assigned by the state licensing agency to assist patients and their families with problems in relation to their nursing-home care. The agencies that can help you with this are listed in the yellow pages under "social service organizations."

299

Will I Have Enough Money to Pay for My Care?

Next to the basic fear of physical dependency, the greatest fear most people experience is the fear of not having enough money to pay for their needs. Being sick often requires expensive care and treatment. If you are too ill or disabled to work, the loss of income, and especially your health insurance coverage, may present an overwhelming financial problem. You can, however, avoid some of the risks by planning ahead and knowing your resources.

Health insurance and Medicare may meet only a part of the ultimate total cost of your care. There are many needs that Medicare does not meet at all, and most private "Medi-gap" insurance policies cover only the 20% "co-payment" of what Medicare does cover.

However, supplemental insurance policies are beginning to offer the kind of coverage that provides for care needs that Medicare and "Medi-gap" insurance do not pay for. If you plan to buy such insurance for yourself, carefully read the sections on limitations and exclusions. Be sure the policy covers nursing-home care at a daily rate level that is realistic for your community. Check that it will cover treatments or care for "preexisting conditions." Some policies have a waiting period for such preexisting conditions, usually three to six months. Others won't cover you at all for any condition that was diagnosed before the start date of the policy.

If you are too sick to work—either permanently or for some extended period—you may be entitled to draw your Social Security on the basis of your disability. If you have dependent children, they would also receive benefits. If you have been disabled for a specified period (as of this writing it is two years), you may be entitled to Medicare coverage for your medical treatment needs. Disability payments are based only on disability, not on need.

If you have only minimal savings and little or no income, the federal Medicaid program can pay for medical treatment and long-term skilled or custodial care. The eligibility rules on assets and income differ from state to state. You should consult your local social services department to see if you are entitled to benefits.

If Social Security benefits are unavailable or insufficient, the Supplemental Security Income (SSI) program is available to those who meet the eligibility criteria for Medicaid.

The social services department in the hospital where you have obtained treatment can advise you about your own situation and the probability of your being eligible for these programs. The local agency serving the disabled usually has advisors who can refer you to programs and resources for which you may be eligible. Senior centers often have counselors knowledgeable about the ins-and-outs of health care insurance.

I Need Help, But Don't Want Help. Now What?

Let's talk about the emotional aspects of becoming dependent. Every human being emerges from childhood reaching for and cherishing every possible sign of independence—the driver's license, the first job, the first checking account, the first time we go out and don't have to tell anybody where we are going or when we will be back, and so on. In these, and many other ways, we demonstrate to ourselves as well as to others that we are "grown up"—in charge of our lives and able to take care of ourselves without any help from parents.

If a time comes when we must face the realization that we need help, that we can no longer manage completely on our own, it may seem like a return to childhood and having to let somebody else be in charge of our lives. This can be very painful and embarrassing.

Some people in this situation become extremely depressed and can no longer find any joy in life. Others fight off the recognition of their need for help, thus placing themselves in possible danger and making life difficult and frustrating for those who would like to be helpful. Still others give up completely and expect others to take total responsibility for their lives, demanding attention and services from their children or other family members. If you are having one or more of these reactions, you can help yourself to feel better and develop a more positive response.

The concept, "*. . . change the things I can change, and accept the things I cannot change, and have the wisdom to know the difference,*" is really fundamental to being able to stay in charge of our lives. You must be able to correctly evaluate your situation. You must identify those activities requiring the help of somebody else (going shopping, cleaning house, for instance) and those activities you can still do on your own (getting dressed, paying bills, writing letters).

This means making decisions, and as long as you keep the decision-making prerogative, you are in charge. It is important to make a decision and take action while you are still able to do so, before circumstances intervene and the decision gets made for you. That means being realistic and honest with yourself.

Some people find that talking with a sympathetic listener, either a professional counselor or a sensible close friend or family member, is very comforting and helpful. An objective listener often helps by pointing out alternatives and options you may have overlooked or were not aware of. She or he can provide information, or another point of view or interpretation of a situation that you would not have come upon yourself. This is part of the self-management process.

Be very careful, however, in evaluating advice from somebody who has something to sell you. There are many people whose solution to your problem just

301

happens to be whatever it is they happen to be selling—health or burial insurance policies, special and expensive furniture, "sunshine cruises," special magazines, or health foods with magical curative properties.

In talking with family members or friends who offer to be helpful, be as open and reasonable as you can be and, at the same time, try to make them understand that you will reserve for yourself the right to decide how much and what kind of help you will accept. They will probably be more cooperative and understanding if you can say, "Yes, I do need some help with . . . , but I still want to do . . . myself." More tips on asking for help can be found in Chapter 10, "Communicating."

Insist on being consulted. Lay the ground rules with your helpers early on. Ask to be presented with choices so that you can decide what is best for you as you see it. If you try to objectively weigh the suggestions made to you, and don't dismiss every option out of hand, people will consider you able to make reasonable decisions and will continue to provide you the opportunity to do so.

Be appreciative. Recognize the good will and the efforts of those who want to help. Even though you may be embarrassed, you will maintain your dignity by accepting with grace the help that is offered, if you need it. If you are truly convinced that you are being offered help you don't need, you can decline it with tact and appreciation. For example, you can say, "I appreciate your offer to have Thanksgiving at your house, but I'd like to continue having it here. I could really use some help, though—maybe with the clean-up after dinner."

If you are at length unable to come to terms with your increasing need to be dependent on others for help in managing your living situation, you should consult a professional counselor. This should be someone who has experience with the emotional and social issues of people with disabling health problems.

Your local agency providing services to the disabled should be able to refer you to the right kind of counselor. The local or national organization dedicated to serving people with your specific health condition (American Lung Association, American Heart Association, American Diabetes Association, etc.) can also refer you to support groups and classes to help you in dealing with your condition. You should be able to locate the agency you need through the telephone book yellow pages under the listing "social service organizations."

Akin to the fear and embarrassment of becoming physically dependent is the fear of being abandoned by family members who would be expected to provide needed help. Tales of being "dumped" in a nursing home by children who never come to visit haunt many who worry that may happen to them.

We need to be sure that we do reach out to family and friends and ask for the help we need when we recognize that we can't go on alone. It sometimes happens that in the expectation of rejection people fail to ask for help. Some people try to hide their need in fear that their need will cause loved ones to withdraw. Families often complain, "If we'd only known . . . ," when it is revealed that a loved one had needs for help that were unmet.

If you really cannot turn to close family or friends because they are unable or unwilling to become involved in your care, there are agencies dedicated to providing for such situations. Through your local social services department's "adult protective services" program or Family Services Association you should be able to locate a "case manager" who will be able to organize the resources in your community to provide the help you need. The social services department in your local hospital can also put you in touch with the right agency.

303

Grieving—A Normal Reaction to Bad News

When we experience any kind of a loss—small ones (such as losing one's car keys) or big ones (such as losing a life partner or facing a disabling or terminal illness)—we go through an emotional process of grieving and coming to terms with the loss.

A person with a chronic, disabling health problem experiences a variety of losses. These include loss of confidence, loss of self-esteem, loss of independence, loss of the lifestyle we knew and cherished, and, perhaps the most painful of all, the loss of a positive self-image if our condition has an effect on appearance (such as rheumatoid arthritis or the residual paralysis from a stroke).

Elizabeth Kübler-Ross, who has written extensively about this process, describes the stages of grief:

- *Shock,* when one feels both a mental and a physical reaction to the initial recognition of the loss.
- *Denial,* when the person tells himself, "No, it can't be true," and proceeds to act for a time as if it were not true.
- *Anger,* the "why me?" feelings and searching for someone or something to blame (if the doctor had diagnosed it early enough I'd have been cured, or the job caused me too much stress, etc.).
- *Bargaining,* when we say to ourselves, to someone else, to God, "I'll never smoke again," or "I'll follow my treatment regimen absolutely to the letter," or "I'll go to church every Sunday," "if only I can get over this."
- *Depression,* when the real awareness sets in, we confront the truth about the situation and experience deep feelings of sadness and hopelessness.

- *Acceptance,* when we eventually recognize that we must deal with what has happened and make up our minds to do what we have to do.

We do not pass through these stages in a linear out-of-one-into-the-next fashion. We are more apt to have several, or even many, flip-flops back and forth between them. Don't be discouraged if you find yourself angry or depressed again, when you thought you had reached acceptance.

304

I'm Afraid of Death

Fear of death is something most of us begin to experience only when something happens to bring us face to face with the possibility of our own death. Losing someone close, an accident that might have been fatal, or learning we have a health condition that may shorten our lives usually causes us to consider the inevitability of our own eventual passing. Many people, even then, try to avoid facing the future because they are afraid to think about it.

Our attitudes about death are shaped by our own central attitudes about life. This is the product of our culture, our family's influences, perhaps by our religion, and certainly by our life experiences.

If you are ready to think about your own future—about the near or distant prospect that your life will most certainly end at some time—then the ideas that follow will be useful to you. If you are not ready to think about it just yet, put this aside and come back to it later.

As with depression, the most useful way to come to terms with your eventual death is to take positive steps to prepare for it. This means to get your house in order by attending to all the necessary small and large details. If you continue to avoid dealing with these details, you will create problems for yourself and for those involved with your situation in a significant way.

The are several components to getting your house in order:

- *Decide, and then convey to others* your wishes about how and where you want to be during your last days and hours. Do you want to be in a hospital or at home? When do you want procedures to prolong your life stopped? At what point do you want to let nature take its course when it is determined that death is inevitable? Who should be with you—only the few people who are nearest and dearest, or all the people you care about and want to see one last time?

- *Make a will.* Even if your estate is a small one, you may have definite preferences about who should have what. If you have a large estate, the tax implications of a proper will may be very significant.

- *Make arrangements,* or at least plans, for your funeral. Your grieving family would be very relieved not to have to decide what you would want and how much to spend. There are prepaid "future need" funeral plans available, and you can purchase burial space where and of the type you prefer.

- *Make a durable power of attorney for health care,* and also one that will let someone manage your financial affairs. (This is discussed in Chapter 12.) You should also discuss your wishes with your personal physician, even if he or she doesn't seem to be very interested. (Your physician may also have trouble facing the prospect of losing you.)

Be sure that some kind of document or notation is included in your medical records that indicates your wishes in case you can't communicate them when the time comes.

Be sure that the persons you want to handle things after your death are *aware of all that they need to know* about your wishes, your plans and arrangements, and the location of necessary documents. You will need to talk to them, or at least prepare a detailed letter of instructions, and give it to someone who can be counted on to deliver it to the proper person when needed. This should be a person close enough to you to know when that time is at hand. You may not want your spouse to have to take on these responsibilities, for example, but your spouse may be the best person to keep your letter and know when to give it to your designated agent.

You can purchase at any well-stocked stationery store a pre-organized kit, in which you place a copy of your will, your durable power of attorney, important papers, and information about your financial and personal affairs. There are forms that you fill out about bank and charge accounts, insurance policies, the location of important documents, your safe deposit box and where the key is kept, and so on. This is a handy, concise way of getting everything together that anyone might need to know about.

- *Finish "business" with the world around you.* Mend your relationships. Pay your debts, both financial and personal. Say what needs to be said to those who need to hear it. Do what needs to be done. Forgive yourself. Forgive others.

- *Talk about your feelings about your death.* Most family and close friends are reluctant to initiate such a conversation, but appreciate it if you bring it up. You may find that there is much to say and to hear from your loved ones. If you find that they are unwilling to listen to you talk about your death and the feelings that you are perceiving, find someone who will be comfortable and empathetic in listening to you. Your family and friends may be able to listen to you later on. Remember, those who love you will also go through the stages of grieving when they have to think about the prospect of losing you.

A large component in fear of death is the fear of the unknown. "What will it be like?" "Will it be painful?" "What will happen to me (after I die)?"

Most people who die of a disease are ready to die when the time comes. Painkillers and the disease process itself weaken body and mind, and the awareness of self diminishes without the realization that this is happening. Most people just "slip away," with the transition between the state of living and that of no longer living hardly identifiable. Reports from people who have been brought back to life after being in a state of clinical death indicate they experienced a sense of peacefulness and clarity and were not frightened.

A dying person may sometimes feel very lonely and abandoned. Regrettably, many people cannot deal with their own emotions when they are around a person they know to be dying and so deliberately avoid his or her company, or they may engage in superficial chitchat, broken by long awkward silences. This is often puzzling and hurtful to those who are dying, who need companionship and solace from those they counted on.

You can sometimes help by telling your family and friends what you want and need from them—attention, entertainment, comfort, practical help, and so on. Again, when a person has something positive to do, they are more able to cope with their emotions. If you can engage your family and loved ones in specific activities, they can feel needed and can relate to you around the activity. This will give you something to talk about, to occupy time, or it will at least provide a definition of the situation for them and for you.

If you choose to die at home, a hospice can be very helpful. These organizations provide both physical and emotional care to people who are dying, as well as for their families. A hospice can arrange for setting up your home to meet your needs and take care of the details of your care both before and at the time of death. This can be a great help to loved ones. To find a hospice near you, ask the hospital social worker, your doctor, or community service information and referral.

Hospice care, as with everything else discussed in this chapter, can be arranged before the time it's needed. Planning ahead can be a comfort to both you and your loved ones.

• • •

Suggested Further Reading

American Heart Association. *American Heart Association Guide to Heart Attack, Treatment, Recovery, and Prevention.* New York: Times Books, 1998.

Barkman, Kip. *The Stroke Recovery Book: A Guide for Patients and Families.* Addicas Books, 1998.

Callahan, Maggie, and Patricia Kelley. *Final Gifts: Understanding the Special Awareness, Needs, and Communications of the Dying.* New York: Bantam Books, 1997.

Copeland, Mary Ellen, and Wayne London. *The Depression Workbook: A Guide for Living with Depression and Manic Depression.* Oakland, Calif.: New Harbinger Publications, 1992.

Kübler-Ross, Elizabeth. *On Death and Dying.* New York: Scribner Classics, 1997.

Kurz, Gary. *Cold Noses at the Pearly Gates.* 1997.

Lewinson, Peter M., Rebecca Forster, and Mary A. Youngsen. *Control Your Depression.* New York: Simon and Schuster, 1992.

Weiner, Florence, Mathew H. M. Lee, Harriet Bell, and Howard A. Rusk. *Recovering at Home after a Stroke.* Body PRC, 1994.

Wilkinson, James A. *A Family Caregiver's Guide to Planning and Decision Making for the Elderly.* Minneapolis: Fairview Publishing, 1999.

CHAPTER
20

200+ Helpful Hints

THERE ARE MANY WAYS TO ORGANIZE YOUR LIFE TO MAKE THINGS EASIER. Necessity, they say, is the mother of invention. If so, then creativity must be the father. Fortunately for us, creative people before us have invented "shortcuts" to make things a little easier for us. Here are a few. These suggestions are offered to jog your imagination and problem-solving abilities. Not everything works for everyone. Use what is helpful.

Waking Up

Try some stretching and strengthening exercises while you are still in bed.

Get a clock radio and set it to awaken you with music rather than an alarm. Some can wake you with a prerecorded tape of your choice. Record the tape with your own "pep talk."

Make half of your bed while you are are still in it. Pull the top sheet and blanket up on one side and smooth them out. Exit from the unmade side, which is then easy to finish.

A quilted comforter and matching pillow cases or pillow shams can replace a bedspread. They are easy to pull up, and carefully smoothing the sheets and blankets underneath is unnecessary, since the thick quilting hides any irregularities in the surface.

Do some of your dressing sitting on the edge of your bed before you get up. Leave the clothes within reach of your bed the night before.

Consider an electric mattress pad for your bed. Turn it on just before you do your exercises to help loosen morning stiffness.

Keep a cane or chair next to your bed to help pull yourself out of bed in the morning.

Bathing and Hygiene

If standing in a shower or sitting down in a tub are too demanding, get a bath stool. It is waterproof and goes right in the tub. You can sit while you bathe.

Shower heads or bath faucets can be replaced with a unit that incorporates hand-held sprayers.

A "sponge bath" can be taken in place of a tub bath and can be a lot less taxing.

If you are weak, don't take a bath or shower unless someone else is at home with you.

A long, absorbent, cotton terry robe will eliminate the effort of drying with a towel.

An oxygen tube can be kept out of the way while bathing by passing it over the shower curtain rod.

Soap on a rope enables you to use soap with one hand, and keeps it from falling.

A liquid soap dispenser may be easier to use than a bar of soap.

If excess humidity bothers you, leave the bathroom door open while you bathe.

Replace difficult twist tops on shampoo or lotions with pump tops.

A shower caddy keeps bathing supplies within easy reach.

Use nonskid safety strips or a rubber bath mat in the tub or shower.

Consider having grab bars installed in your tub or shower to minimize the risk of falling.

Get a long-handled sponge or brush.

Suctioned soap holders make it possible to soap up without grasping the soap or needing to use two hands.

Suctioned brushes are also useful for cleaning dentures with one hand.

Electric toothbrushes and "water pic" appliances make brushing easier.

Get a dental-floss holder if flossing is difficult with two hands.

It is possible to open a toothpaste tube with one hand by holding the tube in the palm of the hand and using the thumb and index finger to open the cap. Use the heel of the hand to squeeze out the toothpaste.

Look for toothpaste in pumps rather than tubes. The heel of one hand can press the pump.

Look for special long and/or curved handled toothbrushes.

Toothbrush handles can be made easier to grasp by wrapping a small sponge or foam hair curler around them.

Ask family members to fold the end of the toilet paper into a "V" to make it easier to grasp.

Have a grab bar or safety frame installed next to the toilet. A free-standing towel rack next to the toilet can also help you when getting off the toilet.

"Le Funelle" or "Sani-Fem" make it possible for women to urinate standing up.

Women who are troubled by occasional accidents of losing urine find that small panty liners or sanitary pads with adhesive backs help avoid potentially embarrassing situations.

Women who find tampons difficult to remove might try winding the tampon string around a pencil and gently pulling with both hands. Some brands have looped strings, making removal with either fingers or a pencil easier.

Women who use pads for feminine hygiene can keep the genital area clean using a squeeze bottle of water kept by the toilet. These bottles can be found with a variety of spray nozzles.

Grooming

A small sponge or a foam hair roller around the handle of a razor or an eyeliner pencil can make them easier to grasp.

Long-handled brushes and combs make is easier to reach hair.

Shaving or applying make-up is easier if you have a low mirror so that you can sit down while doing either.

Talk to a hair stylist about a "drip dry" style. Special haircuts and/or permanents can eliminate rollers and/or hairdryers and still be very stylish.

If you have respiratory problems, switch to nonaerosol toiletries. You can get liquid or gel hair dressings and roll-on or solid deodorants.

Many toiletries can be purchased that are unscented or hypoallergenic.

Dressing

Use the dresser drawers that are easiest to reach.

Lower the rod in your closet or get a closet organizer to bring clothes within easier reach.

It is safer and easier to pull underpants and trousers up when lying flat in bed, if balance or mobility are problems. Graduate to a chair.

Shop for clothes with dressing in mind. Look for easy-to-reach fasteners, front openings, and elastic waistbands loose enough to be pulled over hips.

Look for clothes with Velcro or elastic instead of buttons.

Replace the buttons on your garments with Velcro. Move the buttons to the top part of the opening for decoration.

Bras can be fastened in front and then turned around and pulled into place, or buy front-opening bras.

When putting on pantyhose or a girdle, roll them down from top to bottom, then step in and pull onto your hips and unroll.

Dusting powder on the thighs makes pulling on pantyhose or girdles easier.

Avoid tight belts, bras, or girdles that restrict chest and abdominal expansion.

Avoid tight neck bands. Ties should be loose, or replaced with a bolo or loosely tied scarf or kerchief.

Suspenders (braces) may be more comfortable than a belt.

Put rings or loops on zipper pulls, or get a special "zipper puller."

Many who are bothered by extreme temperatures may find cotton underclothing more comfortable than synthetic.

Use a bent coat hanger, reacher, or "dressing stick" to help with pulling up pants or retrieving clothes that are out of reach.

Most women find that wearing slacks and socks is much easier than struggling into panty hose.

Avoid socks or stockings with elastic bands or garters that may bind the leg and restrict circulation.

Use a "sock donner" to put on socks and stockings.

Get a long-handled shoehorn.

Slip-on shoes are easy and require no bending over to tie.

Convert your lace-up type shoes to slip-ons with elastic shoelaces.

When shopping for clothes, take a tape measure with you that is already marked with your measurements. By measuring the garments, you may not have to try on so many before you buy.

Choose women's pants or skirts with pockets, and carry money, driver's license, and so on, in the pockets instead of carrying a large, heavy purse. A photographer's vest is good for this.

Getting Around

Lead with your stronger leg when going up stairs. Lead with your weaker leg when going down.

Remove all throw rugs—they can cause falls.

Doorways inside your home can be made wider by removing the doors, making them easier to get through with a wheelchair, walker, or other equipment.

Consider installing stair rails on both sides of the stairway to increase safety.

A small ramp can replace a couple of stairs at the entrance to your home or elsewhere.

Carry a folding cane seat with you when you go out. It gives you both something to lean on and something to sit on when necessary.

Look for a walker that has a large basket in front and a small bench seat to sit on when you get tired.

Consider installing a mechanical lift chair on your stairs.

Place a chair or table near the top of stairs for you to lean or sit on when you reach the top.

To lift and carry:
1. Lift or carry while exhaling through pursed lips.
2. Rest and inhale through nose; continue this pattern of intermittent work and rest until you get the job done.

Doing Household Chores

Get a small utility cart . . . some fold, most have at least two shelves. As you move about doing your chores, use the cart to carry your supplies or things that need to be put away. If you live in a two-story house, keep a cart on each level.

Pick-up tongs can retrieve things from hard-to-reach places. The tongs can be purchased from most medical supply houses.

A magnet tied to a string can also help pick up thumbtacks, hairpins, and so forth. It will stick to your cart, refrigerator, or washing machine for quick availability.

Plan your chores so that you go in a circle, rather than back and forth.

Keep a set of cleaning supplies in each area they are to be used to avoid carrying them around.

Long-handled sponges are good for hard to reach areas.

To clean your bathtub, sit on a low stool next to the tub and use a long-handled sponge or clean it at the end of your bath. Then rinse both you and it.

Consider a battery-powered "scrubber" for bathtub, sink, and so on.

Get a long-handled dustbin and a small broom for dry spills. Small brooms can be found in toy stores.

Foam floor mats can be placed where you may need to stand often, such as at the sink, ironing board, or telephone. They can reduce foot and ankle pain and low back pain.

Use an adjustable-height ironing board so that you can sit down while ironing. Attach a "cord minder" to keep the cord out of your way.

Small items such as socks or underwear can be washed in laundry bags to avoid having to search in the washer or dryer.

If lifting heavy detergent boxes is difficult, have someone pour some into a small container, or put a large container on the floor and use a scoop.

For some, a front-loading washer is easier to use than a top-loader.

Use gravity to get clothes out of the dryer or front-loading washer. Put a basket under the door and scoop the clothes into it with a reacher or stick.

Try old-fashioned push-on clothespins rather than pinch clothespins.

Fitted bed sheets are difficult to put on the bed; slit one corner and fasten with a tie.

Use a large, wide spatula or oven shovel to tuck in sheets.

Use a vacuum cleaner with disposable bags, and remove the bag with extreme care, if you have respiratory problems.

A small, battery-powered hand vacuum is easy to use for spot clean-ups and can be kept on your cart.

Those with breathing problems should avoid sweeping and dusting. If you feel you must do it, wrap the working end of the broom or mop with a damp cloth.

A damp cloth is also good for dusting. If you don't want to use anything damp on wood surfaces, get a roll of crinkly paper towels and a bottle of lemon oil. Tear the towels in sections and fold in quarters, put 4 or 5 coin-sized dots of oil on each towel and roll up tight. Store in a zip-lock bag or a jar. Use and discard.

If you must do a dusty job, wear a mask.

Have good ventilation and an adequate supply of fresh air at all times.

People with respiratory problems should observe the "no aerosol" rule for cleaning products.

Avoid harmful substances that can vaporize, such as mothballs, solvents, and kerosene.

Put lockable casters on furniture you wish to move to clean around.

Cooking

Microwave and convection ovens save time and energy.

Replace the twist-ties on bread or other foods with clothespins.

Avoid lifting heavy pots of food along with the water they were cooked in. Place food in a basket to lower into the water for cooking, or get a spaghetti cooker provided with a perforated insert. You can lift the basket out to drain food. Someone else can drain the pot later, or you can ladle it out.

Ask family members not to close jars too tightly. A jar opener can be mounted under a countertop, or you can get a rubber disk to help you open jars.

Try to replace any heavy cast-iron or ceramic utensils with lightweight pots, bowls, and dishes.

317

Don't try to get everything done at once. Almost all jobs can be divided into small tasks. For instance, clean the top shelf of the refrigerator today and the bottom shelf tomorrow.

Plan your meals when you are neither hungry nor tired. Light, well-balanced meals are too important to leave to impulse.

A number of small meals is better than large ones, especially for a person with limited lung capacity, to allow more room for lungs than for the stomach.

Use convenience food when desired, but remember that many packaged foods have high salt and sugar contents. Read the labels.

Keep plenty of water in the refrigerator. You can get containers to sit on your shelf that have spigots near the bottom so that you won't have to lift the container to fill your drinking glass.

For many recipes, it's just as easy to cook double or triple quantities as small ones. Freeze the excess in meal-sized containers and enjoy some cook-free meals when you feel like a day off. In a microwave, they can be easily thawed and heated without drying out.

A slow-cooker or crockpot can make many meals easier to prepare, as can a pressure cooker.

Always use an exhaust fan when cooking, especially if you have respiratory problems.

A small, portable fan can help you overcome shortness of breath from exertion or cool you off in a warm kitchen or laundry room. Some are battery-powered and can clip on a shelf or counter.

Use your cart when tidying up after a meal. For example, gather all the items that need to go into the refrigerator, and then sit down with the cart and put them away all at once.

Put your most used pots and pans back on the stove and leave them there. Instead of putting dishes and silverware away, reset the table for the next meal.

Try a cutting board with spikes sticking up that will hold meat firmly in place while you cut it. If necessary, you will be able to carve meat with one hand.

Select appliances with levers or pushbuttons that are easy to operate.

Store canned goods so that the same items are lined up behind one another. Storing them upside-down allows you to see the labels more easily.

Get attractive cooking pots that double as serving pieces.

Disposable foil pie tins, loaf pans, and so on, save clean-up effort.

Line pans with aluminum foil for easier clean-up.

Get pans with nonstick surfaces for quicker clean-up.

Stabilize mixing bowls by placing them on a wet washcloth or by placing them in an open drawer at work height.

Put flour and sugar in conveniently located containers so that you won't have to lift the heavy bags.

Oven mitts allow you to lift hot pans with both hands.

Use a bent coathanger or a dowel with a hook on the end to pull out hot oven racks.

Attach a spray hose at the kitchen sink, and fill pots with water while they sit on the countertop or stove.

A pizza wheel can cut more than pizza easily!

A small food processor can make short work of grating, chopping, or slicing.

One or two wheeled stools in the kitchen will make work easier . . . at counter height or low enough to allow you to get into lower cabinets with minimal bending.

Eating

If you have difficulty using a knife, try a "rocker knife" or pizza cutter, which require the use of only one hand.

Use a scoop dish with a nonskid bottom to avoid shoving food off of the plate.

Boating supply stores are a good source for stable, nonskid dishes.

For easier grip, build up utensil handles with pieces of foam and tape.

Entertaining

Buffets are easy. Let guests serve themselves.

Party supply stores have very attractive and festive disposable plates, utensils, and serving pieces.

Plan a potluck rather than doing it all yourself.

Dessert potlucks are especially popular.

Buy two tickets for an event and ask a friend.

Remembering Medications

A pillbox with a separate compartment for each day of the week is useful. A pill-box like this can be made out of an egg carton or purchased at your pharmacy.

Take-out food places often have 1-oz plastic containers for salad dressing and ketchup that can be labeled and used for each pill-taking occasion during the day.

Some electronic pillboxes can be programmed to "beep" you when it's time to take your medication.

Combine your medication-taking with a normal, daily habit, such as brushing your teeth or watching the news. Put your pills next to the things you use for that activity (making sure your medications are out of the reach of children).

Whenever you get a prescription filled, figure out how long it will last and mark the time to reorder on a calendar. This may save you from running out in the middle of the night or on a weekend or holiday.

Shopping

Find grocery stores and pharmacies that deliver, or buy on the internet.

If you are shopping with an oxygen carrier, find a shopping cart on your way in and put the oxygen in it while you shop.

When you are grocery shopping, have all the perishables packed in a separate bag. When you get home, put them away and leave the rest for later.

Some supermarket chains are now offering motorized, riding shopping carts.

Community service clubs and churches will sometimes offer shopping services for people with disabilities. Volunteers will shop for you.

Mail-order catalogs offer just about everything you would want and are fun to look through, too. You need only to be able to plan ahead a little.

If you have a home computer with a modem, you can do a lot of shopping by computer.

Order stamps through the mail or on the internet..

Going Out

Get assertive about exposure to other people's tobacco smoke. You have a right to breathe smoke-free air. Ask smokers near you to stop.

Wash your hands well when you get home. Colds and other diseases are often spread by touch.

Find out where you can get a daily air-quality report for your area and use it when making your plans for the day.

Before going out, prepare for your homecoming. Lay out your comfortable clothes and slippers, leave a drink in a handy thermos, set out whatever utensils you will need for your evening meal, even turn down your bed. Homecoming can then be a real relief.

321

If you don't already have one, ask your doctor about getting a handicapped parking permit. Even if you don't drive, a friend can use this when you go places together.

If you will have to sit in the car for a long period of time, make up a kit of helpful things such as a pad and pencil, paperback book, tissues, and so on. A coffee can with a snap-on plastic lid can be an emergency urinal.

If you must fill the gas tank, get upwind so that you don't inhale the fumes.

If you worry about being away from a phone in an emergency situation, consider a mobile phone.

When shopping for a new car, look for easy-to-open doors and easy-to-adjust seats.

Attach a loop to the inside door handle of your car to make it easier to pull closed.

Wide angle rear-view mirrors allow for increased visibility without straining your neck.

A back support device (such as Sacro Ease) can make a car seat more comfortable.

Gardening

A riding mower, preferably with a self-starter, can be a real morale booster.

Find lightweight, easy-to-handle tools. Many tools now come in lighter, durable plastic.

Use a folding stool or one with wheels. There are wheeled stools especially for gardening, with a tool storage area under the seat.

Many tools can be purchased with a long handle, or you can have a short handle replaced with a long one.

Build up planting beds so that you can sit on the edge and garden.

Enjoying Recreation and Leisure

If you like to play cards, try a card holder.

Get to know your neighbors. Think of a signal, such as a pulled down shade at night, to let them know you are OK.

Start a buddy phone system. Regular calls to and from friends are good for you, and these contacts will be able to aid in case of an emergency.

Somewhere near you, there is someone who needs your friendship and help, too. Look for these opportunities.

You can play board games long distance by mail, over the phone, or by computer.

Home computers and Web TV are getting more and more reasonable to own. Many games, including card and board games we all grew up with, are now available for home computers. You can have your own "Wheel of Fortune" game, with music and color graphics, right at home.

Your computer can also introduce you to other people by e-mail.

Learn to use your computer or take art classes in an adult education class in your community. Your mind needs exercise, too, and you can meet interesting people in class.

Many adult education classes are offered through television or correspondence.

If you find your previous hobbies too demanding, try scaling them down for the time being. Start a container garden or try bonsai or orchids rather than a full-sized garden, for example.